MAINE STATE LIBRARY

WITHDRAWN

joseph j. bean, jr. MERCY HOSPITAL
rene laliberty MID-MAINE MEDICAL CENTER

decentralizing hospital management

A Manual for Supervisors

▲▼ **ADDISON-WESLEY PUBLISHING COMPANY**
Reading, Massachusetts ■ Menlo Park, California
London ■ Amsterdam ■ Don Mills, Ontario ■ Sydney

658.91   B367d   1980   copy 1

Bean, Joseph J.

Decentralizing hospital
management :
        MAINE AUTHOR

Library of Congress Cataloging in Publication Data

Bean, Joseph J.
    Decentralizing hospital management.

    Includes bibliographical references and index.
    1. Hospitals—Administration.   2. Hospitals—
Personnel management.   3. Supervision of employees.
I. Laliberty, Rene, joint author.   II. Title.
RA971.B34   658'.91'3621   79-25159
ISBN 0-201-00556-5

Copyright © 1980 by Addison-Wesley Publishing Company, Inc. Philippines copyright 1980 by
Addison-Wesley Publishing Company, Inc.

All rights reserved. No part of this publication may be reproduced, stored in a retrieval system,
or transmitted, in any form or by any means, electronic, mechanical, photocopying, recording,
or otherwise, without the prior written permission of the publisher. Printed in the United States
of America. Published simultaneously in Canada. Library of Congress Catalog Card No. 79-25159.

ISBN 0-201-00556-5
ABCDEFGHIJ-AL-89876543210

foreword

H.R. Hornberger, M.D., Mid-Maine Medical Center, Waterville, Maine

Known in the literary field as
Richard Hooker, author of M*A*S*H

Asking me to write a foreword to a book about hospital administration may be a little like asking Leo Durocher to say nice things about umpires. I don't know how to run a hospital. I've always avoided involvement in the business and management areas of medicine. I've justified this by proclaiming that I have a full life just trying to be a reasonably competent journeyman surgeon. My exposure to medical administrators has been limited to semiannual tirades when I get mad about something, pick on the first administrative type I run into, and call him or her bad names. Despite my height of 6'3", I find that with increasing age and girth, this technique has lost some of its effectiveness. I begin to fear that some seemingly sleeping midget may become annoyed with me to the point of doing something about it.

I don't presume to be able to evaluate all of this book. Much of it is as far beyond my comprehension as the techniques of pneumonectomy is beyond the authors'. We're working in the same business with different but indispensable talents.

The business of decentralizing hospital management is a concept I'm not even sure I understand because I do not understand anything said to me by hospital administrators, lawyers, or auto mechanics. What I think the authors are saying is that each unit of an organization should be run by someone who knows how to run it. This reminds me of a ward in my hospital that, for the first nineteen years of my practice, was run by a nurse who knew how to run it. She had no fancy nursing education, but she knew what was going on in her ward. She functioned, in a rural hospital with no interns or residents, as a nurse, an administrator, an intern, and a senior resident. If I wanted to avoid responsibility on a Saturday or a Sunday, I could call this lady and say, "Have I gotta come in?" There were three possible responses: (1) Yes, Doctor, you should come in and see Mrs. Jones. (2) No, Doctor, it's all clear. (3) I'm concerned about Mrs. Smith, but if you'll let me know where you'll be, I'll call you if I'm seriously concerned.

Now that this lady has retired, the same ward has the same number of patients, three times the personnel, and if you call in, about the best you can get is the patient's height, weight, color, temperature, and blood pressure. This amounts to name, rank, and serial number, which adds up to no confidence that the people in charge are doing more than going through the motions.

This may be a digression, but I think I see the same deterioration of intelligent responsibility in all clinical areas. Obviously, this is my area of interest, and my interest extends to wishing that each area of the hospital could be run by competent people who are not so overcome by the overall administration that they fear to function as individuals.

I do know something about two of the major interests of the authors, which are "cost containment" and "caring." I know that folks at the administrative level have to be concerned with cost containment, but I was surprised at their understanding and clear definition of the need for "caring" in the medical industry.

As for "cost containment," I know something about this but not much. We have an explosion of technical gadgets, and they save and prolong lives that were routinely lost twenty years ago. The gadgets cost tens and hundreds of thousands of dollars. Does the cost justify the results? The answer is an unqualified "yes," but the public can't comprehend this and the politicians comprehend nothing. Technology has advanced to the point where, if we don't use it, we are vulnerable to malpractice suits. Therefore, we overuse it, often against our clinical judgment but for self-protection. There is no way hospital management can contain these costs.

Recently, just before leaving on a two-week vacation, I saw a patient who had complaints virtually diagnostic of cancer somewhere in his belly. I referred the patient to an internist with the recommendation, "Get somebody to crack him open and save time and money."

The internist just called me. He said, "The diagnostic workup cost the State of Maine three grand but showed nothing. Then we operated and found a cancer of the cecum. I should have taken your advice." If he'd taken my advice and found nothing, he and the surgeon would have been accused of unnecessary surgery performed without adequate preoperative workup.

The legal profession has a large responsibility for the skyrocketing cost of medical care. Hospitals and doctors have to pay exorbitant insurance rates for malpractice insurance. I recently said to a high official in the Department of Health, Education and Welfare, "You guys are laying it on us to contain costs, but you'll do nothing to get the lawyers off our backs."

His answer was, "The lawyers make the laws. They're more responsible for inflated medical costs than you guys, but we can't do anything about it."

Decentralizing Hospital Management has pleasantly surprised me by discussing at length the subject of "caring." At all levels of medicine, it's easy to forget to be nice. The busy surgeon who has three seriously ill patients in the Intensive Care Unit may be curt with the wife of a "routine gallbladder" who needs two minutes of time but wants ten. The guy mopping the floor may be impolite if a half-blind eye patient ignores the "Caution" sign he has posted to warn of a slippery floor. At the physician level, it's still possible for the sincere, concerned incompetent to achieve greater material success than the genius who forgets that every fascinating, intellectually stimulating problem belongs to a scared human being. Too often, the genius either will discuss the problem in terms the patient can't possibly understand or will be brutally honest, an increasing tendency resulting from a variety of factors and theories I disagree with.

Decentralizing Hospital Management emphasizes the importance of putting the patient at ease and showing consideration from admission to discharge. Every year at the Mid-Maine Medical Center, where I and a coauthor work, we have, in summer, many patients from out of state. We also have patients the year round from outside our immediate area. A week seldom goes by without a patient saying to me, approximately, "I've never been in a hospital like this before. Everybody has been so nice."

I have noticed, however, as our organization has grown, a small but perceptible diminution of this personal touch. I have long suspected that we hire more and more people to do less and less and that some of these people would do better in a car wash. No matter how thoroughly something has been explained to some patients, they'll ask a nurse's aide questions they forgot or were afraid to ask the doctor. I would like to have some of the authors' group commanders indoctrinate the aides. Recently a patient of mine, in for an operation she knew had some risk, was told, "Oh, yes, most of them do well, but he did lose one, right in the next bed."

This is the kind of "care" the patient doesn't need. This patient, a former nurse, told me the story on her first postoperative office visit. "Why didn't you tell me before?" I asked.

"I was afraid you'd get mad and try to wipe out the administration, and I wanted all your attention." Some of these patients *are* thinking.

Decentralizing Hospital Management is a valuable contribution to the mechanics of health care. Doctors, particularly those like me who are totally disinterested in hospital administration, should put it on their reading lists.

preface

In the health care field today, there is now great interest in such areas as rising payroll costs, wage/salary administration, performance evaluation, job evaluation, communications, supervisory development programs, and so on. Much of it is not advancement and development of management thinking, but pure reaction to the threat of bureaucratic control and to other external pressures, public, social, and economic. Hospitals are beginning to recognize that they must begin improving their basic management skills if they are going to survive under some of those pressures!

The health care industry today is concerned about its current managerial effectiveness, and rightly so. They are beginning to realize that, as health care providers, they may not be totally in command of things in the years ahead.

The complexity of modern-day hospitals is now starting to be recognized; the inadequacies of many people in administrative, department-head, and supervisory positions is also becoming more apparent. It is also becoming obvious that the only effective way the cost spiral can be checked is through a cooperative team effort, relying on effective and efficient supervisors. There are thousands of recorded adjudicated cases of inadequate patient care in hospitals where there was no deficiency in technical and professional competence. But because of ineffective and inefficient supervision resulting from improper planning, inadequate organization, lack of understanding of basic management techniques, lack of coordination, and the absence of programs of measurement and control, competent professional employees were poorly motivated and unable to perform, and patients did not receive the quality of care to which they were entitled. Or the quality was there but delivered at an excessively high cost. Or the quality and cost were within an acceptable norm, but the delivery was effected in an uncaring, uncompassionate manner.

Productive, efficient, and loyal workers must have effective and efficient supervisors. There are identifiable reasons why some hospitals are effective while others do poorly. Faced with the challenge of providing a multitude of expanded health care services of higher quality at a lower cost in a caring, compassionate manner, while operating in an inflationary economy, the health care institution can meet the challenge only through the development of a supervisory staff that fosters favorable employee attitudes toward the patient, the public, the job, the department, and the institution.

The health care field is beginning to experience a supervisory development that has been prevalent in the industrial sector for decades. Progressive health care administrators are beginning to acknowledge that management as a science cannot be confined to the "administrator's office," and that effective supervision is an art and a science that needs to be coupled to all technical disciplines if an institution is to grow and prosper. These facts are important from both the human and the technical sides of management and administration in profit-making and nonprofit enterprises, including the private and public sectors.

Portland, Maine   J.J.B.
Waterville, Maine   R.L.
January 1980

acknowledgments

Special thanks to John A. Sheridan of John Sheridan Associates, Inc., Des Plaines, Illinois, and to W. I. Christopher, President of W. I. Christopher & Associates, Inc. (now a subsidiary of Modern Management Methods, Inc., Bannockburn, Illinois), 17 Hortense Place, St. Louis, Missouri, for their technical support and authorship of Chapters 2 and 3, respectively. Also to Gerald W. Fuller, Fellow of the Hospital Financial Management Association (FHFMA), Vice President of Finance, Mid-Maine Medical Center, Waterville, Maine, for his exceptional chapter (Chapter 4) on "Marketing of Hospital Resources." Thanks also to Michelle Hallee from the Personnel Department staff of the Mid-Maine Medical Center, who carefully assimilated our manuscript and kept us on schedule to meet the publisher's deadline requirements. She also finalized the manuscript, assisted by Jane Wheeler of the Personnel Department staff of Mercy Hospital, Portland, Maine.

We are deeply indebted to H.R. Hornberger, M.D., Mid-Maine Medical Center, for his Foreword, which added a unique new dimension to our book, to Linda LaVerdiere, R.N., Physician's Assistant, Mid-Maine Medical Center, for her intermediary accomplishments, and to Mary Jane Geer, Health Information Specialist, Mercy Hospital, for researching and providing much background material.

We would like to acknowledge and express our gratitude to Clarence R. Laliberty, Jr., Administrator of Miles Memorial Hospital, Damariscotta, Maine, for his confidence and support and for allowing us to field-test some of our manuscript material over a six-month period at that hospital.

A special thanks to Gerald M. Homer, Administrator, Old Bridge Regional Hospital, Old Bridge, New Jersey, for his contributions (especially to Chapter 5) while he was a member of the Maine Society for Hospital Personnel Administration.

Our appreciation to Eugene Beaupre, M.D., President of the Mid-Maine Medical Center, and Howard Buckley, Executive Director of Mercy Hospital, for encouraging and supporting our efforts.

As you can see, many have helped in our writing efforts, and our acknowledgments would not be complete without a nod to Jeffrey G. White, Vice President of Operations at the Mid-Maine Medical Center. As chairman of its Caring Environment Committee, he breathed life into a program that was viewed by many as an impossible objective.

authors' comments

Effective and efficient health care delivery is today more dependent than ever on the quality of supervision at all levels. The term "supervisor," as it pertains to the contents of this book, in intended to embrace all those individuals whose duty it is to function as those members of management having the authority, in the interest of the hospital, to affect the flow of work in their departments, or to direct employees in the daily exercise of their duties.

Effective and efficient management needs an informed supervisory staff. Business and industry have for decades relied heavily on their supervisors and have recognized them as an integral part of the management function. Modern, progressive management in hospitals is also beginning to recognize that service is provided and work is performed through people. Good employer–employee relations are more than ever dependent on good supervision, and the supervisor at all levels is the "key" man or woman in the organization who must assume the responsibility for that important role and its sweeping implications. The hospital supervisor today is faced with the challenge of providing more service, of higher quality but at a lower cost; in addition, supervisors must be cognizant of the fact that the services are delivered in a manner that projects the hospital as a caring humanitarian institution. This goal can be accomplished only through the development of a supervisory force of the highest caliber.

Perplexing, complicated problems face today's hospital chief executive officer in ever-increasing numbers. Not the least among them is the issue of cost containment. Cost containment is a major concern facing the entire health care industry. As more and more pressure is brought to bear on the health care industry to curtail escalating costs, it behooves those in hospital supervisory positions not to overlook cost-containment elements within their respective departments. Recognizing this, we have pinpointed areas in this book that show the greatest potential for cost containment within a health care institution.

It is our hope that this manual will highlight and clarify topics within the realm of management and will assist hospital supervisors in implementing some cost-containment programs within their areas of responsibility.

Citizens in metropolitan areas are viewed as indifferent and uncaring. Their cities are perceived by people from rural areas as unfriendly places to visit. The health care industry is being accused of this same seemingly unfriendly behavior. The medical staff must share that criticism along with the hospitals. To deal with the image problem, hospital supervisors must understand the basic causes of the public's widespread loss of faith in our health care delivery system. It is important that hospitals change their public image. The attitude of all employees in all departments toward their jobs, their departments, their hospital, and the public they serve must be favorable. An effective and efficient supervisory force is one that develops and maintains a caring environment within the institution.

This book has been planned and designed to assist the supervisor in acquiring the basic knowledge, skills, and attitudes needed in the modern management of a health care institution.

Joseph J. Bean, Jr.

Rene Laliberty

contents

Whether hospitals will survive as free-standing institutions or become bureaucratic public-service agencies is going to depend on the degree to which supervisors are able to effectively manage their departments, the degree to which the industry learns to control its cost, and the degree to which the industry is humanized. The ultimate solution to health care effectiveness and efficiency is decentralization of hospital management.

maintaining a caring environment

What other objectives should a health care institution have beyond that of providing beds and progressive health care services? A fast, and frequently the most common, answer is "What else should we be doing?" Some may respond by saying that our concentration should be on continually expanding objectives related to the multiplicity of services provided to the community. Those sharing this position also suggest that the expansion of health care technology, coupled with increases in costs, cost controls, and the additional work force required to deliver these new services, will consume most of the available financial resources, precluding the possibility of any additional endeavors. From the standpoint of economics and practicality, proponents of those views are correct in their observations. The health care industry should be commended for its technical and medical progress. However, the industry must also be admonished for its shortsightedness in failing to recognize that while these services to the patients are a hospital's primary objective, they can no longer be its only objective. The health care industry has too long allowed itself the luxury of objective apathy. It has allowed and tolerated tunnel-vision setting of objectives—all under the guise of a public service being performed and all else being secondary. It has forgotten that humanism is as important as professionalism.

Although there is no statistical proof available within the active beehives of many hospitals, health care is indeed delivered in a perfunctory manner. While there are no official documents on the subject, many individuals will attest to the fact that care was delivered to them as former patients in an uncaring manner, lacking in human compassion. It appears, then, that while our standard objectives and intentions are realistic and appropriate for a health care institution, our delivery and salesmanship are inadequate and are being challenged by the public we serve. We are at a point where the patients we are committed to, care about, care for, and try to help are saying, "Your charges are too high," and "I'm not being treated with compassion." Whether hospitals will survive as freestanding institutions or become just another public service, such as a post office, city hall, or government agency, is going to depend on the degree to which the health care industry learns to control its costs and the degree to which the industry is humanized and perceived as such by the public.

The dilemma is not limited to health care institutions. Private physicians frequently treat the public, both in the hospital and in their offices, with as uncaring an attitude as is displayed within the hospitals by some hospital personnel. Frequently, the patient's out-of-pocket dollars for a doctor's office visit purchase the professional services of a nurse rather than those of a physician. It is only fair at this point to emphasize that indifference and disrespect are not confined to hospitals and physicians—they are quite common throughout our society at the present time.

For some reason, the public will tolerate some surliness from store clerks and taxicab drivers but will have a significantly lower tolerance level when a health care professional exhibits a similar attitude of indifference. Much of the service provided by hospitals is for relief of pain, anxiety, or disability. Because the measurable and technical elements of patient care are beyond the understanding of most patients, their assessment of service received centers on factors such as convenience, friendliness, and comfort.

Doctors frequently "set the tone" in relationships with patients. Nurses and others directly associated with "hands-on" patient care who observe confrontations between physicians and patients are not going to be inspired to make an effort to be friendly and courteous. It needs to be said that while there are instances of uncaring physicians on every staff, there are also numerous compassionate doctors who set a caring example. There are also many who are unaware that their behavior is anything but exemplary, and they need only to be reminded by their colleagues that the welfare of individual patients is served more effectively if harmony and proper attitudes are displayed.

Aside from the traditional hospital functions of patient care, continuing education, care evaluation, and physician rounds, a caring-environment function must be added as a hospital's primary objective if the health care industry is to fulfill the demands and expectations of the American public.

There's something highly contagious about a hospital that practices the art of "humanization." It's not a bug, not a virus. It's a warmth of feeling, a compassionate way of dealing with people. It's the kind of atmosphere that generates unsolicited return letters from patients, such as the following:

> When you enter a place, your first impression is usually the lasting one. Naturally, patients are going to be apprehensive; but if they are greeted in a friendly way—with a smile—it helps soften things so one doesn't feel so nervous and upset.

> Well, I was one frightened woman—I won't say girl, because I'm 74 years old—when I came to your hospital. Everybody was marvelous, from the man who fixed my bed with traction to the doctor who left his home late at night and stayed with me until I was up in my room. Nobody could have cared more—and they've followed through in the same spirit up to the last minute while I was in your hospital for four weeks.

> With people who are hurt, or sick often, you get a kind of panic . . . to us it's serious and it's frightening. A simple explanation is all it takes . . . it helps us to relax.

The X-ray people were gentle and did everything possible to help me. It wasn't easy handling me. Nobody could have been kinder.

I'm in my seventies, and I'd never been in a hospital before. I never saw the inside of your hospital until two weeks ago. I never knew what the nurses did, what the doctors did, or a single thing. Well, now I know, and your hospital is a credit to the town and to the people.

I've been in and out of hospitals most of my life. I've been in hospitals all over the world, but I prefer yours because it has a heart.

Just being able to talk to someone can help them more sometimes than giving them an injection.

They even gave me the recipe for that wonderful seafood chowder.

A current and popular belief in the health care field is that the responsibility for projecting and protecting the hospital's image as an efficient, effective, and caring institution is the job of those in administration. In a world that seems lacking in human concern, the hospital as a symbol of caring remains uppermost in the minds of the public. Frequently, the cold institutional feeling is inadvertently communicated to the patient, which angers him or her since it contradicts the image of the hospital as a place that "really cares." To the patient, the hospital seems disorganized and hurried. The result is that the health care professional is viewed as an anonymous person, at times performing unexplained procedures that have no relationship to the immediate needs of the patient. Instead of getting a feeling of being served, he or she gets the feeling of being either managed or ignored.

Many communities take great pride in their hospitals and periodically survey the public for their impressions. Actual letters from one such survey cause one to reflect and ask, "Is the task of projecting and protecting the hospital's image really only the administration's responsibility?"

Unless one is rushed in (out cold or gasping for life), the Emergency Room is just another waiting room—noisy and smoke-filled.

I believe in recent years the government programs have enabled the hospital to expand at a greater rate than is feasible, and everything is becoming larger and more impersonal with no increase in the quality of patient care.

Long waiting hours in emergency rooms or clinics is definitely no good. As you see, I need help.

Thank you for the good care I got when I got it.

Explain why the patient is ill, not just give them pills to keep them quiet and out of the way for more patients and more money.

We brought our son in with a possible leg fracture, and he was asked if he could hop to the desk to sign papers.

Your patient billing is so fouled up the patients have no idea how to handle it.

I have been left lying naked and cold with no bath blanket around me, while the L.P.N. ran to the kitchen to get a certain food list for the patient beside me instead of finishing my bath.

They do not know what the word "compassion" means.

The faults I find with your hospital are largely those of increasing inefficiency and thoughtlessness.

Last winter I visited a dying 80-year-old woman at your hospital. It seemed wrong to me that on the last day of her life she had to be bothered by loud music coming over the PA system.

Why do patients almost always have dinner and all meal trays set on the over-bed table when the urinal and toilet paper are still there?

The heart is gone from the hospital.

Feel you've lost considerable ground on the caring side of medicine.

Your nurses are too indifferent towards their patients.

The hospital is now a big business. It's lost its individual personal interest in compassionate care.

Dr. Eugene M. Beaupre, a practicing physician and President of the Mid-Maine Medical Center, Waterville, Maine, has for many years been a patient-relations advocate, prescribing the caring aspect of health care as part of the total process of our health delivery system.

His efforts and philosophy of total patient care are appropriately reflected in his often-repeated statement:

> The physicians and their plan of treatment for a patient are only part of the total care program. We, as hospital employees, must reach out and convince the patients by our actions and deeds that we do indeed care for them as people. The maintenance of a positive attitude towards not only the patient but our fellow employees will minimize many of the uncaring horror stories directed towards the health care industry. Hospitals must reestablish an atmosphere so that each person within the institution understands that the prime goal of the institution is to create and maintain a humanitarian caring environment which stresses the emotional and psychological well-being of the patient as well as the patients' physical needs. A hospital's patient care and human-relations environment are composed of the aggregate of all employees' attitudes. Those in a supervisory capacity have a responsibility to help each employee appreciate his or her contribution and to identify with the goal of the institution. There are six common courtesies that, if practiced, will make the balance of the prescription for a caring environment a simple routine:
>
> - always call patients by name;
> - introduce yourself to patients as you would like to be addressed;
> - explain what you are going to do in terms the patient can understand;
> - smile;
> - be gentle; and
> - have respect for the feelings and needs of other members of the hospital family.

Many subtle messages are transmitted in the first five minutes after a patient arrives at the hospital for admission. The following suggestions are for those involved in the admitting process, showing how they should act during those crucial 300 seconds.

- Be there when the patient arrives and greet him or her warmly. The admitting office or desk that is unoccupied is communicating to the prospective patient, "So what if you're here, I'm busy right now, I'll get to you later."
- Look professional and be well groomed. The message you want to convey by being appropriately dressed is that you are a preview of

the dress standard to be expected from others during the patient's stay.

- Share some social or casual conversation with the patient. You can cement the bond in a very real way. This shows you want to know him or her as an individual, not just as someone who came to occupy a bed.
- Be responsive to the patient's mood. If you detect nervousness or apprehension, respond in an uncritical, sympathetic way to dramatize that you're really concerned about his or her feelings.
- Don't place the preparation of your admitting papers above everything else. Complete your questionnaire as casually and as quickly as possible.
- Escort the patient to the room. Introduce him or her to the responsible person on the assigned unit. Don't leave the patient alone in the room, and be sure there is someone there to carry through with the second phase of the admitting procedure.

"Good employee morale" and "esprit de corps among the work force" are often mentioned as being ideal factors that constitute, or contribute significantly toward, the effectiveness and efficiency of an organization. Certainly these are needed and one cannot minimize their importance. However, in a hospital setting other factors are necessary before the institution can be viewed by the public as truly effective and efficient. Patients can sense whether the attitude of those they come in contact with is totally positive. Employee attitudes should be considered and viewed as a significant segment of a patient's care plan. Feelings and attitudes of the hospital staff are important, not only for the institution's morale index but also for the patient's progress and well-being. Employees who are ill-tempered, poorly motivated, or unhappy will more than likely be rude and display an uncaring attitude to both patients and the public. The feelings generating from the hospital's staff can be counterproductive for the patient and can be a significant contributory factor depicting the hospital as "just another institution."

Each department, depending on its function, may want to adopt varying codes of conduct for employees. The following code, adopted by a head nurse in a medium-sized rural hospital in the Northeast, is indicative of some of the guidelines that can be communicated by a hospital supervisor to employees.

- Keep in mind the fact that your voice may greatly affect the nervous system and the emotions of others.
- Speak in a gentle, firm tone, and avoid leaving the impression of aggression, whining, drawling, or jitteriness.
- Avoid idle chatter, gossip, shoptalk, and self-centered topics.

- Refrain from entering into or prolonging a conversation when you are angry or emotionally disturbed.
- Be respectful in conversations, including the use of names and titles.
- Start the conversation with a patient when you recognize that his or her condition and mood warrant doing so.
- Do not pour out your own personal history and problems to the patient. The patient may seem interested, but the story of your life will not hasten recovery in the least. In listening, the patient becomes the nurse.
- Avoid talking too much or too little, and appreciate the therapeutic value of being a good listener.
- Remember that your conversation and actions impress patients, and this impression causes them to form opinions about you and the hospital.
- Professional appearance and personal grooming are of vital importance, and patients expect them to be above reproach.
- Remember that patients tend to absorb fears, anxieties, tensions, and conflicts from their surroundings.
- Exert patience, tolerance, and understanding with patients and visitors.
- Carry out physician orders accurately and sustain confidence in the doctor and all members of the health team.
- Respect the religious beliefs of patients.
- Treat the patient's family and friends with kindness and friendliness.

Most people who work in hospitals think of doctors as independent and undisciplined individuals living in the lap of luxury and riding around in Cadillacs. Some physicians may well deserve or earn such a depiction; however, they are in the minority and the image should not be applied to all doctors. There are many who sacrifice financial gain, time, and comfort to help the less fortunate. As a rule, most physicians value their independence and abhor interference and regulations. Supervisors and health care employees could save themselves a great deal of frustration if only they would attempt to know and understand the value structure of their medical staffs. For one thing, physicians are not employees of the hospital. A doctor's primary loyalty is to his or her patient and not to the hospital. Supervisors frequently fail to recognize this and expect the physicians to adhere rigidly to all hospital policies. Moreover, the doctor does not always have to be in control. However, those who say that the physician is never going to be in control are ignoring the realities of hospital organization. Organizationally, the doctor is not the boss; functionally, however, the doctor must be the boss. Hospital employees must be able to recognize and accept those differences if they wish to maintain human-relations harmony within the hospital setting.

There are those who propose that a patient advocacy program is very effective toward resensitizing the hospital staff to the primary reason for its existence—that is, to serve patients well. There is equally strong opposition expressed among health care workers to a patient advocacy program, which they see as a stumbling block, promoting only ambivalence and paranoia among the staff. In certain instances a patient, directly or through a representative, may express dissatisfaction or voice a complaint that cannot be resolved via normal channels. From the patient's point of view, then, the patient advocate is a means of expressing that objection or having questions resolved. However, most of those involved in the health care system view the advocate as nothing more than a positive listener, friend, supporter of patients' rights, and ultimately, an ineffective catalyst for resolving issues. The effectiveness of patient advocacy by itself as a means of maintaining a caring, humanitarian environment in a hospital setting is questionable. Conflict or competition between departments in a hospital is a very common situation; therefore, it is doubtful that any one person or program can possess all of the requisites necessary to be effective. Patients do not have much influence in hospitals, and a patient advocate who stands alone and attempts to give the patient a voice in hospital matters has little chance of survival. A patient advocacy program can be successful only if it is part of, and closely linked to, an overall institutional objective of developing and maintaining an ongoing humanitarian, caring environment.

The public's demand that hospitals control and be held accountable for their costs does not overshadow its appreciation for quality care and concern. A recent editorial in a daily Northeast newspaper sums it up rather well:

> Hospitals aren't San Juan Sheratons or Miami Marriotts, but you could have a smashing Caribbean vacation for what it costs to stay in one.
>
> That's the way it seems, at least, when you pay (or more likely send to your insurance carrier) the bills that result from a few days visit at your local hospital.
>
> Somehow, though, you don't feel a bit like complaining at that stage. You got a lot of attention from some very skilled and compassionate people when you needed it. You wouldn't have wanted any corners cut to save money.
>
> It seems clear that the people who run modern hospitals have sought to make hospitals as nearly fail-safe as is humanly possible. That takes a lot of people and a lot of money.
>
> A recent surgery patient counted at least nine people

with whom he was directly involved between the time he entered the lobby and the time he got to the room that was to be his dwelling place for the next five days. Most of them were charged with assessing his physical condition to determine what was necessary to get him through the experience successfully.

He was aware of at least ten people (in addition to two accomplished surgeons) who were involved in getting him to, through, and away from the surgery for which everything else had been prelude.

Countless other men and women fed, washed, and otherwise pampered the recovering body during the days and nights of surgical postlude that followed.

There may well be some redundancy in all of this. It might be possible to eliminate some of the steps and cut costs with a relatively small increase in risk to the patient.

However, our recent patient found it both comforting and reassuring when, seconds after he coughed unexpectedly in the middle of the night, a flashlight appeared at the foot of his bed and a soft voice asked, "Is everything OK?"

The first step toward the development of a caring environment is for the hospital Governing Board to adopt a resolution stating that it endorses and is directing the hospital staff to develop a humanistic health care delivery system as one of its primary objectives.

In a decentralized hospital management situation, the department head or supervisor then must accept the responsibility for instilling and maintaining within his or her areas of accountability an atmosphere conducive to promulgating and furthering that objective. However, without a plan of action, it is impossible to translate concept into reality. The following is a recommended course to follow on a departmental or unit basis.

- Orient the staff to their responsibility.
- Communicate to employees that the "caring-environment concept" is going to be an ongoing objective.
- Conduct a departmental audit or assessment to identify procedures, facilities, practices, and attitudes that are counterproductive.
- Outline a plan to correct or improve negative results found in the audit or assessment.
- Outline a plan to expand on the positive results from the audit or assessment.
- Solicit suggestions from employees for programs needed to strengthen job satisfaction.
- Follow up and implement some of the employee suggestions.

- Communicate the aims and objectives of the program frequently.
- Display a genuine caring attitude for employees.
- Communicate positive employee actions.
- Conduct a telephone courtesy campaign.
- Encourage top management to regularly visit your employees and work areas.
- Review and enforce dress codes.
- Review and enforce smoking policies.
- Involve, where appropriate, volunteers and medical staff members in the action plan.
- Check patient waiting areas for cleanliness, orderliness, and privacy.
- Include aspects of maintaining a humanitarian, caring environment as part of the probationary evaluation report on new employees. A sample evaluation report (Exhibit 1-1) can be found at the end of this chapter.
- As part of the employee annual evaluation process, include an addendum related to the objective. A sample addendum (Exhibit 1-2) can be found at the end of this chapter.

Hospitals are on the firing line from many sectors of our society today for many reasons. Some of the criticism is justified; much of it is not. Not all of the criticism is amenable to corrective action, but that which has to do with the humanism of hospitals can be readily addressed. However, corrective measures must begin within the system, and the only people that can substantially effect those measures are the hospital's first-line supervisors. Consumers of the nation's health care industry are no longer silently wishing that things were different—they are loudly demanding that their criticisms be heard. For both ethical and pragmatic reasons, hospitals are well advised to respond to the consumer demand for humanism in their institutions and to advise supervisory staffs to ensure that the response is carried out at every level of patient care.

EXHIBIT 1-1

EVALUATION REPORT ON NEW EMPLOYEE

Name: _____   Dept.: _____

Job title: _____   Probationary period ends: _____

Date employed: _____   Evaluate not later than: _____

Return to Personnel Dept.
not later than: _____

	POOR	AVERAGE	GOOD
QUANTITY OF WORK Consider volume of work expected of a new employee.	____	_____	
QUALITY OF WORK Consider accuracy of work; also spoilage, errors, or mistakes.	____	_____	____
DEPENDABILITY Attendance, promptness, etc.	____	_____	____
ATTITUDE Consider relationships with patients and personnel, i.e., courtesy, tact, cooperation, etc.	____	_____	____
INITIATIVE AND APTITUDE FOR JOB Consider acceptance of responsibility; ability to follow and retain instructions, etc.	____	_____	____
SAFETY HABITS Employee's attitude toward safety rules and regulations.	____	_____	____

The prime goal of the hospital is to create and maintain a humanitarian, caring environment that stresses the emotional and psychological well-being of the patient as well as the patient's physical needs. "Caring" goes beyond direct patient care areas—kindness and courtesy toward all with whom we have contact is a vital part of everyone's job. The hospital's patient care and human-relations environment is comprised of the aggregate of all employees' attitudes. Therefore, those in a supervisory capacity (especially during the evaluation process) have a responsibility to help each employee appreciate his or her contribution and identify with the goal of the hospital. Our goal is to create an atmosphere in which employees can feel a high degree of self-esteem and in which the level of patient care is high.

Exhibit 1-1 (continued)

Have you informed the employee that the *prime goal* of the hospital is to create and maintain a caring environment? _____

Do you believe the employee personally accepts and will work toward the attainment of this goal? _____

Have you informed the employee that our performance evaluation process includes factors relative to his or her effectiveness in assisting us to maintain a caring environment? _____

Our orientation program stresses the importance of six common courtesies: (1) always call patients by name; (2) introduce yourself to patients as you would like to be addressed; (3) explain what you are going to do in terms the patient can understand; (4) smile; (5) be gentle; and (6) have respect for the feelings and needs of other members of the hospital. How consistently does this employee project these courtesies? _____ Always. _____ Improvement needed. If improvement is needed, has this goal been established with the employee? _____

Remarks by dept. head or supervisor: _____
_____
_____
_____

Remarks by the employee: _____
_____
_____
_____

I recommend that this employee be: retained _____ .   **released** _____ .

_____   _____
Signature of employee   **Signature of department head**

_____   _____
Date   **Date**

EXHIBIT 1-2

ADDENDUM TO THE PERFORMANCE EVALUATION REPORT
(For use in annual reviews)

The prime goal of the hospital is to create and maintain a humanitarian, caring environment that stresses the emotional and psychological well-being of the patient as well as the patient's physical needs. "Caring" goes beyond direct patient care areas—kindness and courtesy toward all with whom we have contact is a vital part of everyone's job. The hospital's patient care and human-relations environment is comprised of the aggregate of all employees' attitudes. Therefore, those in a supervisory capacity (especially during the evaluation process) have a responsibility to help each employee appreciate his or her contribution and identify with the goal of the hospital. Our goal is to create an atmosphere in which employees can feel a high degree of self-esteem and in which the level of patient care is high.

Please consider, discuss, and comment on these factors when you evaluate each employee. Return this addendum form with the regular performance evaluation form.

1. Have you informed the employee that the *prime goal* of the hospital is to create and maintain a caring environment?_____

2. Do you believe the employee personally accepts and will work toward the attainment of this goal? _____ How? _____

_____

_____

3. How effectively does the employee function in personal contacts required by his or her position? (Consider tact, courtesy, self-control, and judgment in relations with patients, visitors, fellow employees, and others.) _____

_____

_____

_____

4. How effectively does the employee communicate with others? (Consider telephone use, giving directions or assisting visitors, oral expressions, and written expressions.)_____

_____

_____

_____

5. How effectively does the employee function in human-relations situations with the medical staff, residents, and fellow employees? (Consider negativism, willingness to help, respect for others, discretion, etc.) _____

_____

_____

Exhibit 1-2 (continued)

6. Does the employee project a favorable image of a person employed in a health care institution? (Consider dress standards, gum chewing, smoking or eating in public access areas, etc.) _____

_____

_____

7. Our orientation program stresses the importance of six common courtesies: (1) always call patients by name; (2) introduce yourself to patients as you would like to be addressed; (3) explain what you are going to do in terms the patient can understand; (4) smile; (5) be gentle; and (6) have respect for the feelings and needs of other members of the hospital. How consistently does this employee project these courtesies? _____ Always. _____ Improvement needed. If improvement is needed, has this goal been established with the employee? _____

_____

What efforts have you recommended to the employee for self-improvement? ____

_____

_____

When will you be reviewing these self-improvement efforts with the employee? ____

_____

Does the employee have suggestions that should be considered to improve the hospital's caring environment? Please specify. _____

_____

_____

_____   _____
Signature of employee   Signature of department head

        _____   _____
                Date   Date

2

the
supervisor
and
decentralization

(This chapter was written at the special request of the authors by John A. Sheridan of John Sheridan Associates, Inc., Des Plaines, Illinois)

> "Labor can do nothing without capital; capital nothing without labor, and neither labor nor capital can do anything without the guiding genius of management; and management, however wise its genius may be, can do nothing without the privileges which the community affords."

This statement of W. L. MacKenzie King's was made in a speech before the Canadian Club in Montreal in 1919. Like most rhetoric, it ties everything into a neat bow but at the same time leaves loose ends.

This chapter will elaborate on some of those loose ends and will also address the subject of a supervisor working in a centralized or decentralized environment.

First off, what is suggested by the term "supervisor?" What do we do when we "supervise?" Mainly, we oversee, direct, or *manage* work, workers, or a specific project. In any definition of supervision, we are bound to trip over the words "manage" and "manager." These words are like reformed hookers: their past is much more interesting than their present.

The word "manager" comes from the Italian word *maneggiare*, which originally meant to train (a horse) in its paces. Anyone who has attempted to manage can appreciate the analogy between a balky and stubborn horse and a recalcitrant worker.

If we asked a rank-and-file worker, "What does your supervisor *do* every day?" just what would that worker say? Probably, in the simplest possible terms, that a supervisor tells other people what to do. The supervisor is, in fact, the *boss*.

Other worker expectations are that the boss will kick us in the ass if we get out of line, will take a straight party line with "upper" or "senior" management people on most issues ("*they* are always right; *we* are always wrong"), will "snitch" on us if given half a chance, and will give us an occasional bribe in order to quell a riot or bleed one more foot-pound of work out of our already fatigued bodies. Finally, we expect the boss to pay us on time and accurately.

These expectations are easy transferences from the educational system that produced these workers. Back in high school and maybe even as far back as grade school, there was an authority figure who confirmed all these same expectations. Sometimes it was the principal, at other times the administrator, and at still others the teacher. However, it is becoming difficult to view the teacher as an authority figure when he or she carries a picket sign.

In business and industry, there is even a report card, the paycheck we receive for having "passed." Presumably, if we don't get paid, we have "failed."

My profession, labor relations, forces the participants in the daily Divine Comedy of Business to hone and fine-tune the definition of a supervisor or manager into subtle shades of difference. This continually forces the question "What is a supervisor?"

Most of the time, the question is posed as a direct by-product of the confrontation between labor and capital. Usually, these confrontations take the form of labor disputes, i.e., union-representation election campaigns, strikes, walkouts, job actions, "sick-ins," "sick-outs," and, in short, the entire bevy of diabolical ways that workers have devised to withhold their labor and rest their fatigued bodies awhile.

Since 1935, labor relations in this country have been regulated by a body of law known as the National Labor Relations Act, "as amended." The blood of this law was the Wagner Act, passed in 1935; the sinew came later, in 1947, with the passage of the Taft-Hartley Act.

This law is enforced on a daily basis by a much maligned but, in many ways, quite traditional federal agency known as the National Labor Relations Board. Over the years, the "act" and the board have had a great deal to say in answer to the question "What is a supervisor?" Sometimes what they have had to say has been a non sequitur, but then, one might expect that one of the oldest federal administrative agencies would set the pace for all the others.

It is important to note that managers' thinking about how they will organize to do business, what their organization chart will look like, how many levels will be in the pyramid, who will carry what job titles, and what to do about many other decisions has been and will continue to be done within the context and the setting of the National Labor Relations Act, as well as being guided by the rulings of the National Labor Relations Board.

For instance, suppose that you and I are going into partnership to form a new company. We plan to manufacture and bottle "Inflation Repellent." For this important enterprise, we estimate that we will need about eighty production workers. Using a one-to-twenty ratio, we also figure that we will have four "supervisors." However, we decide that we will call three of these supervisors "leadmen" or, in post-1964 parlance, "leadpersons," and only the fourth will be called "supervisor" or some other such appellation befitting the lofty rank involved.

Why have we chosen to call these three "leadpersons"? First, as good capitalists, we want to get the most out of everyone. By calling them leadpersons, we reckon that we can keep them on the time clock at an hourly wage, exclude them from the management benefit package (which may include an annual trip to the Galapagos Islands, in order to field-test the Inflation Repellent), and most important, require them to spend a certain amount of their time performing exactly the same duties performed by the rank-and-file workers.

As part of our management plan, we have also decided to forgo a third partner—the AFL-CIO—in all its pomposity. In other words, we don't want a union in our shop.

By creating the category of leadperson, we have already laid a minefield for the unwary and unsuspecting union that is lurking outside our door. If and when the union shows up, circulates its authorization cards, and files a petition for an election with the National Labor Relations Board, these mines will explode into a form of gas known as "lawyer's verbiage." This gas will manifest itself throughout the record of the NLRB hearing, as well as in many supporting documents, exhibits, briefs, and even in the final decision of the Regional Director who rules on our case.

Throughout this hearing procedure, which one industrial-relations director of a famous eastern tool-manufacturing company calls the "mating dance of the storks," will run one continuous thread—one oft-repeated question—"Are they *supervisors?*"

Why is the answer of any consequence? Because if the board decides that they are indeed supervisors, they will not be allowed to vote in the impending election. On the other hand, if the board decides they are not supervisors, they will be allowed to vote. Elections can be and have been decided by such rulings, and it is impossible to determine just how many megaliters of gas have escaped in the pursuit of such pithy points.

Supervisors, not surprisingly, are not covered by the "act." They may form unions, but management does not have to recognize them. Consequently, in the jungle of the workplace, they really have no rights other than those poured onto them from that great eyrie known as "senior management." To quote MacKenzie King once again:

> Management, however wise its genius may be, can do nothing without the privileges which the community affords.

Of course, the expectations of the average employee concerning a supervisor ("kicks us in the ass . . . straight party line . . . snitch . . . bribe . . . pay us on time . . . etc.") are all dolled up by the NLRB when they attempt to define a supervisor's duties, but when the "uptown" clothes are stripped away, it all comes out the same.

The NLRB wants to know if the supervisor can hire, fire, promote, demote, give money, take it away, etc. If these clothes don't fit, they also ask if our supervisor can, at a minimum, *effectively recommend* any of these things. I have italicized "effectively recommend" because that is precisely what this chapter is really about. "Effectively recommend" poses this question:

> "Does anybody listen to what the supervisor has to say on these matters, and *act* on the information he or she has provided?"

Over the years, it has been my experience that this question is asked not only by the NLRB; more often than not it is also asked by the supervisor!

AUTHORITY, CENTRALIZATION, AND DECENTRALIZATION

> Be not afraid of greatness: some are born great, some achieve greatness, and some have greatness thrust upon them.
>
> *Twelfth Night,* Shakespeare.

Many years ago, I was a union organizer in Chicago. As an organizer, I spent many hours holding fifteen-cent beer aloft in one hand while pushing union authorization cards with the other. One day, in one of my favorite gin mills on the West Side, I noticed the following sign over the bar:

> Three weeks ago I couldn't even spell supervisor . . . now I are one!

This bit of folk wisdom is an accurate reflection of what sometimes happens in the real world of business and industry. It also forces us to consider seriously the question "Where do supervisors get their authority?" Just what is the ineffable "something" that makes one person work for another?

Classically, in the American industrial setting, supervisors have risen from the ranks. By dint of hard work and a bit of luck, the best bottler in our mythical Inflation Repellent plant — we'll call him Joe — rises, after a good deal of trial and error, to become supervisor of the bottling line. It is important to note that most of the reasons Joe gets the job have little or nothing to do with managerial skill (training the horses in their paces?) or administrative ability.

If lucky, Joe will function awhile in the "halo effect" of his informal group. This means that as a worker he was a popular and trusted member of the clique, perhaps the *most* popular and trusted member. If so, he was an *informal leader.* Informal leadership is the very best kind, since it is conferred on us silently and tacitly by our peers. No election takes place, no ballots are marked, no polling occurs; people simply follow him because he has "command presence."

Unfortunately, this halo effect has a half-life and soon goes by the boards. After all, the newly appointed supervisor has deserted the clique that was "home" for so long and has gone over to the side of the "enemy" — the *management,* also known as "them." At this point, to demonstrate the required competence, Joe needs help, and that help can come from only one source — his senior management.

It is appropriate to ask, "What kind of company do "they" (Joe's management) want Inflation Repellent, Inc., to be — centralized or decentralized?" The answer is critical, since it will affect our supervisor's every waking hour.

In a decentralized organization, authority will be consciously and willingly distributed from its main center (the "top") among and toward its widest parts (the "bottom"). On the other hand, in a centralized organization, it will be jealously kept within a core group, usually at the apex. Either approach is bound to have the most far-reaching effects on how people are supervised.

About 20 years ago, our firm represented a gray-iron foundry in a midwestern state. It employed about 300 people who were involved in producing toilets and their appurtenances. There were 15 supervisors, but we soon learned that they were "supervisors" in name only. Stories abounded of employees who reported to work drunk, were discharged by their supervisors, and then went to the plant manager's house and, by telling a sob story, gained reinstatement the following day. This could certainly be called a "centralized" environment. It could also be called lousy management.

Another story bears telling. A small, family-owned packaging firm was headed by a president who was having a tussle with the demon rum. At one point, he was absent from the premises for over a year, first on a prolonged binge and then in the arid plains of a detoxification center. Who was in charge during his absence? Since Nature abhors a vacuum, the plant functioned, and profitably, because of a tenuous detente between the line supervisors and certain members of the informal organization, the "hidden" leaders. This is the best example of *total* decentralization that my pen and memory are able to muster.

Oddly enough, both of these situations produced the same symptomatic result, that is, a long and traumatic union campaign. In the first case, the company lost by one vote; in the second, the company won by about 2 to 1.

In *both* cases, by seeking union representation the employees were giving their managements the same message, loud and clear: *The union will get this place organized.* Although it may seem redundant to say that "being organized will get us organized," this message was implicit in the means chosen by the workers, which is, after all, the only means they have available. To quote McLuhan, "The medium is the message."

In the setting of labor relations, there is a "damned if you do, damned if you don't" quality to the "centralize or decentralize" debate. Consider the problem of the banking industry as it ponders the specter of unionization.

Since 1967, unions have shown an interest in organizing the employees of banks and other financial institutions. Most large commercial banks present a "one bank" facade to the public. Nothing could be further from the truth. A large commercial bank is highly specialized and decentralized. It has many separate divisions such as Trust, Commercial Lending, International, Retail Banking, etc. A brief discussion of retail banking will focus on the serious labor relations implications of the centralization versus decentralization question.

One of my clients has a retail banking division composed of hundreds of consumer branches, spread over a large metropolitan area. Until recently, this division had been operated in a highly centralized fashion. This simply meant that all meaningful decisions had been made "downtown" rather than "out there in the boonies."

A new executive was placed in charge of this division, and he brought a philosophy of decentralization with him. In his first meetings with subordinates, he told them that "branch managers would run their own business," and that "each branch would be an autonomous profit center—totally accountable for its own performance." This executive was not embarking on a laboratory experiment to test theories he had learned in business school. He was, in fact, attempting to improve the previous lackluster performance of the branch system—to make more money at the "bottom line" than had been made in the past.

As his labor relations consultant I watched nervously, but as a businessman I watched with a sense of admiration. My nervousness was based on my knowledge that as he placed each brick of his decentralized scheme in place, he weakened the bank's argument for one voting unit of all employees in the branch system, or—at the very least—all employees in a region of the system, should the day ever arise when a union decided to organize. My admiration came because I knew in my heart that a decentralized system would probably result in a better-managed and more profitable branch operation.

What are some of the criteria used by the NLRB to decide whether the voting unit should be the "great big system" or the "little single branch"? Here they are, in "laundry list" fashion.

1. The extent of the centralized control of the commercial and administrative aspects of the business
2. The extent of the geographic separation of the particular unit being petitioned from other units in the operation
3. The extent of the employee interchange among the units
4. The amount of personal contact between employees of the units (in other words, the extent to which personal contact is limited strictly to the employees of the particular unit)
5. The extent of centralized or decentralized control of labor policy (including not only where the overall level of wages and fringe benefits is determined, but also where other working conditions of real importance to employees are determined, such as decisions on hiring, individual increases, promotion, discipline, and the like)

Seemingly, if one wanted to avoid having the union "carve out" a small, single-branch voting unit, all one would have to do would be to design a company that met all of the criteria listed above, i.e., lots of centralized control of the business and personnel, maximum personal contact and interchange of employees, and minimal geographic separation. We know from experience, however, that this is not always possible. Business lives in the very real world of competition. What may be good labor relations is not always good business.

When the banker in my example tells his branch managers that they are "autonomous," that they will be "running their own business," he opens the way for a union to divide and conquer by picking up, piecemeal, separate units of the operation.

To illustrate, many years ago our firm handled a union campaign for a large New York insurance company. The union showed up at the company's data-entry operation, which was located across from a shopping center on Staten Island. There were about 72 employees, and 8 others were classified as supervisors or managers. On its initial hand-billing effort, the union was able to sign up about 60 of the 72 employees. Forthwith it filed a petition for an election, to be held in the Staten Island operation alone and in no other. The employer had three other operations where employees performed identical work—two on Long Island and the largest in Manhattan at the home office. The employer and his attorneys quickly reasoned that if they could expand the unit to include these other three units, the union would have to either obtain sufficient additional cards or retire *hors de combat*.

When I first interviewed the management and described the NLRB criteria, there was absolutely no question in their minds that they met all of the criteria for a large unit rather than for separate smaller units, of which the Staten Island unit was one. They believed, for instance, that all personnel matters were administered centrally, and that there was interchange of employees from one location to another and personal contact as well. Since the location was a stone's throw from the end of the Verrazano Bridge, they felt that geography was no problem. "It's close to us here in the home office." Imagine their surprise when, after three months of legal machinations, they lost their case, and an election was held among the 72 employees on Staten Island. I had foretold this result shortly after my first visit to the Staten Island facility. As I approached the building, I noticed a "Help Wanted" sign prominently displayed in the front window, which faced the shopping center. When I asked the manager of the facility about this sign, he said, "We get a lot of walk-ins out here. We hire them and send the paperwork into New York."

That branch manager was innovative in other ways as well. When I noticed that we were the only people in the building on that Friday morning and inquired as to the whereabouts of the employees, he winked and said, "Let's have a little secret that New York doesn't know about yet—we have a *four day week* out here. It's an experiment."

Rather than bore the reader with the entire checklist, it was soon apparent that the company had a weak case for centralization and the union had a strong one for decentralization. There was almost no interchange of employees between Staten Island and the other satellite units, and there was no personal contact between the employees of those units.

Somewhere along the way, someone in senior management had told this branch manager that he was "in charge"—that he was the "boss"—and by God, he took them at their word!

From a purely practical viewpoint, labor relations aside, a decentralized company faces other problems as well, mostly in the area of communications. A friend of mine is at the head of the largest single unit of a worldwide publishing empire. His unit is composed of nine separate entities; the company as a whole has about eighty units, composed of dozens of entities. Each day, he is faced with this conundrum: "How do I manage my unit so as to function as a completely autonomous profit center, without going off the deep end and running counter to the goals, objectives, and philosophy of the corporation as a whole?"

Naturally, in this setting, one would expect that the corporation would make these goals, objectives, and philosophies abundantly clear through first-class communications, both written and oral. Unfortunately, this is not always the case, and when the choir begins to sing, they sometimes find themselves singing from different hymnals. According to my friend, the separate and diverse divisions of this well-known company often find themselves so at odds with one another that it seems as though one's corporate brethren are really one's competitors.

When the employees of this division recently completed an attitude survey, they gave my friend a message—loud and clear: "To hell with the parent corporation! Why don't they leave us alone and allow us to 'do our own thing'?" It was obvious that his employees had "bought into" the concept of decentralization and autonomy, so much so that the parent had come to be viewed as an irrelevant nuisance that bled profit off the top for its own ends.

Consultants, especially those dealing in labor relations, are frequently asked to comment on the advisability of a centralized or decentralized course. A labor consultant who tells you, as a manager, that the centralized course is always best is speaking from a narrow professional viewpoint, without regard to doing business. Doing business in the most profitable mode should be your first consideration. Good labor models can always come later.

Let us return to the New York insurance company for a moment. Originally, the company had all its eggs in one basket, in a single data-entry operation located in New York City. The people in management felt that such concentration left them vulnerable. What would happen, someone asked, if a union ever organized that single unit and took it out on strike? They then reasoned that the best defense against such a

single-unit work stoppage would be to erect a number of satellite operations in and around the New York area. Such operations were set up in
short order; one of them was the Staten Island branch previously
referred to. All would have proceeded swimmingly had the Staten
Island manager understood (1) that he had no authority, (2) that all
decisions of a commercial and of a personnel nature were to be made
centrally in New York, (3) that a high degree of interchange of employees was desirable, and (4) that a maximum amount of personal
contact of employees should take place. In other words, the company
was designing a centralized model against the arrival of a union so that
all of the units together would be deemed appropriate for purposes of
collective bargaining, thereby making it virtually impossible for any
union to penetrate the larger group.

Life just doesn't work that way. Not only didn't the Staten Island
manager understand that this was the model, but also he was operating
under the impression that he was responsible, on his own recognizance,
for the day-in and day-out operations of the Staten Island facility, with
only slight regard for overall corporate policies and procedures. It is
reasonable to assume that any comparably motivated self-starter who
had been given a first big managerial assignment within this company
would have acted in exactly the same manner.

Moreover, his actions must be viewed within the context of one
particular division of the whole company, namely, Operations. That
division was well known for allowing its managers to run on a "longer
leash." Therefore, an already motivated manager found himself operating in a freewheeling environment, where his aggressiveness could
be nurtured and run rampant.

The sorry outcome of this story was that the manager was penal-
ized for having the first union drive in the history of the company, and
even though the company won the election, he was later transferred to
a minor position where he now has little or no authority. So much for
the rewards offered by American business and industry to one who, in
the words of a typical Wall Street Journal ad, "is a self-starter, a man
who can think on his feet, who is bottom-line oriented, etc."

In any given year, my firm handles around 100 unionization
attempts on behalf of employers. A unionization campaign has the
following seven stages.

1. In the "restless natives" stage, something is afoot but the employer
   does not quite know what. Only rumors and "rumbles" come to
   the surface.
2. The union appears. Its representatives may telephone and ask for
   an audience with the president. They may write a letter. They may
   demand recognition as the bargaining agent for the employees,
   without the nicety of an election.

3. The union files a petition with the NLRB for an election.
4. A hearing, sometimes formal, sometimes informal, is held ("mating dance of storks").
5. A decision and direction of an election is issued (the world at large learns from the arcane depths of the NLRB who can and can't vote and when the election will be).
6   The election is held.
7. The results are certified.

Our firm is usually called somewhere between stages 1 and 3. When we are called on to assist, we are more or less given carte blanche; in fact, nothing is too good for us. On occasion, we have been offered the client's airplane, his pied-à-terre—everything short of his wife (there have been occasions when I believe that he would have willingly thrown her in, too!).

Many times, these panicky clients have been surprised to find that all we require is control of the supervisory organization for the weeks up to and including the election. Thus begins the greatest exercise in managing by decentralization—a well-run and smoothly functioning union election campaign.

As we meet the supervisory group, we find them a towering mass of Jello. They are afraid; they are nervous; they are intimidated; they are unhappy, bordering on malevolent. In short, they are reflecting all the grievances and complaints of the workers they supervise. Our job is to shape this towering mass of Jello into an effective team that will function, at least on a short-term basis, as a "Swat Force" with one objective in mind—protecting the company from encroachment by the union.

To accomplish this objective, we begin by meeting with the company's supervisors and giving them a basic labor relations orientation. Although the apparent purpose of this orientation is to cover the "do's and don'ts," that is, the legal and illegal aspects of the compaign, there is a more subtle purpose. At this early juncture, we must convince them that they will be totally responsible for the outcome of the election— win or lose. We are merely their consultants—their counselors—and we will share our expertise with them for the duration of the "war." It is they who will go out on the field of battle (the factory floor, the hospital cafeteria, the retail marking room) and carry the message.

At first, there is skepticism. They have heard this before from their own management, only to find themselves ignored or bypassed. Besides, they think, how will we (the consultants) ever know whether or not they (the supervisors) are doing an effective job of campaigning?

The answer is very simply, that we will keep track. We will, in fact, design a feedback system that will continually tell us:

1. what we should write in our campaign letters;
2. what effect our letters and our campaign, in general, are having on the voters;
3. who in supervision has the worst (read "pro-union") departments;
4. who in supervision has the best (read "pro-company") departments; and
5. how the election will come out.

Frequently, we are able to predict the outcome of the election within five percent just by paying close attention to supervisory feedback. In this setting, is it any wonder that we are able to motivate supervisors to carry the message, especially when they know that after the election they will be held accountable for the result?

To digress for a moment, how would one run a centralized campaign where all of the communications came from the top, with little or no supervisory involvement? I am reminded of an election we handled for a company in the Midwest. The particular plant under petition was a branch operation of a West Coast firm. It had a local superintendent who reported to the corporate central offices in Oregon. Prior to our arrival, the corporate offices had retained a local labor attorney without regard to the wishes of their local manager. Early in the campaign, after we had been retained, the local manager came in and showed me a letter from the attorney, which went something like this:

> Dear _____ ,
>
> I am sending, under separate cover, six posters that I have found to be effective in other union campaigns. Post these in a conspicuous place, one per week, between now and the election.
>
> Under no circumstances should you involve your line supervision in the campaign process. It has been my experience that such people are usually ignorant and will inevitably bring down unfair labor practices on the company's head.
>
> Very truly yours,

Such a campaign, if it had been conducted, could certainly have been characterized as "centralized." It also would have failed. We, of course, recommended that the attorney be fired and that one be retained who knew something about labor relations.

In a decentralized campaign, supervisors are allowed, even encouraged, to design their own campaign, to make decisions, to plot strategy and tactics—in short, they are compelled to become involved, to be committed, and to participate.

Let us say, for instance, that our side (the "good guys") decides to pass out a letter to employees during the union campaign that explains our fringe-benefit program. This communication would be managed in the following fashion.

1. The supervisors would be called together as a group and asked for their thoughts on what the letter should say.
2. The letter would then be written.
3. The supervisors would be called together again, and the letter and its contents would be reviewed with them. They would be asked for questions, comments, and criticisms. (Often, the letter is changed because of this meeting.)
4. The letter would be passed out by the supervisors on a one-on-one basis. Supervisors would be told to discuss the letter and to seek conversation, questions, reactions, etc.
5. Supervisors would then be called in and asked, one by one, to recall individual reactions, questions, etc. These reactions and questions would be very carefully recorded.

It is by the above method that the management is able to judge the true feelings of its employees about the union during a union campaign.

Each and every written communication is carefully managed in the same fashion. Nothing is left to chance. All reactions are recorded. In time, it dawns on the supervisors that someone is listening to them —paying close attention to what they are doing and saying. They are, in fact, *accountable.*

Frequently, we are asked why this can't be the case during "peace-time" periods, that is, at times when the company is not under attack by a union. The answer seems to be that, on a daily basis, managers are loathe to delegate the ongoing and continuing authority necessary to run a truly decentralized operation. Only when they are in trouble do they turn to their line or "primary" supervisor (often referrred to with contempt as "the lowest level of supervision," as if they were speaking of some type of household germ.)

It was, is, and always will be a truism in labor relations that for the purposes of communication, the primary supervisor is the key link between top management and the rank-and-file employee. This fact holds true in both centralized and decentralized settings, but it is easier to achieve through decentralization.

You and only you can decide how you want to do business at Inflation Repellent, Inc. I hope you will make the right decision.

3

the hospital
supervisor
as a
decision maker

(This chapter was written at the special request of the authors by W. I. Christopher, President of W. I. Christopher & Associates, Inc., St. Louis, Missouri)

The unwilling often fear the unclear, the uncertain, or the unknown. When all events occur as planned there is no problem, but when changes either planned or unplanned occur there is need for a decision. This often places the hospital supervisor in a predicament. When the options are not clear, the decision or choice of option can be a most difficult proposition. There is often a sense of urgency, prompted by some person who is waiting for directions on how to proceed. The supervisor reluctant to render a decision hampers the whole operation. There is a need to discern the several appropriate choices to be made, and there is then the need to make that choice.

MISCONCEPTIONS ABOUT DECISION MAKING

Any supervisor is aware of the problems created when higher levels of management fail to render an appropriate and timely decision. All the frustrations of the supervisor are equally borne as frustrations by the employees when the supervisor fails in this decision-making process. In many situations the supervisor labors under many misconceptions about decision making, such as the following.

1. Because of the service-oriented concept of management—recognition of the fact that the management, in effect, serves the employee, and not the old belief that the employee serves the management—there has traditionally been the practice of looking to higher levels of management to solve problems and render decisions. As a result, one major misconception is that decisions are made at the highest level of the organization. This is not true. Each level has an appropriate pattern of decisions that must be made and, in fact, are constantly being made in some manner.

2. Because of the pressure of any given situation, another misconception is that the one in charge is responsible for making the decision. This is also not true. Since the impact of participative management and the implementation of MacGregor's "Theory Y," it is not only possible but often desirable that the concerned group be involved with the one in charge when exploring the various options and arriving at an appropriate decision. This process often ensures minimization of resistance and resentment, and creates acceptance of and a commitment to the decision of the group.

3. There is often the untrue belief that a supervisor has responsibility but lacks authority, and that decision making requires authority. One is delegated authority, and in the acceptance of that authority, one creates responsibility. Therefore, the supervisor has specific

responsibility, with authority to render decisions appropriate to that level in the operation.

4. At times the uncertainty of outcome may prompt the supervisor not to make a decision. In effect, to decide not to decide is a very vital decision. However, this decision tends to impede progress, handicap performance, and retard the achievement of the desired results.

It seems important, then, to examine not the problems but the process of realistic decision making.

THE RIGHT TO ACT AND AN ABLE RESPONSE

Nobody in an organization has the right of independent action. Structural authority—that authority delegated to one within the framework of the organizational structure or system—is in fact the delegation of the right to act in a specified manner. This always comes from one's superior. It is not delegated freely and without restriction. One may receive the right to act without restriction, which is full authority. It is more likely that one will receive the right to act and report, the right to act on consent, or the right to act on consent and report. In each situation the right to act is related to a specific task or action. Once authority is delegated, it is the responsibility of the superior to verify that it has been accepted. In the act of accepting authority, workers impose on themselves the instant creation of responsibility, which can be expressed simplistically as the ability to use the right to act in a specified way.

In the process of delegating authority, two issues immediately arise. The first is a belief that one has authority and, therefore, one can exercise it at will. The more autocratic or authoritarian the operation is, the more likely that this belief is true. In democratic processes, however, another issue arises. That issue is recognition of the fact that actual authority is what has been delegated, but operational or functional authority is the amount of actual authority that one's subordinates would permit one to use. Thus the importance of the relationship between the superior and the subordinate is identified. The united or collective action by the subordinates can, in fact, negate the exercise of authority by the superior. In other words, the supervisor can exercise authority only so long as the workers are willing to accept that authority, which is usually expressed to the employee as a decision. The supervisor, in turn, is delegating authority to the employee to act or to perform actions in a specified way, and when the employee accepts that authority there is again the creation of responsibility. This process creates a network of partnerships. As authority is delegated away, since one cannot delegate it and still keep it, one creates a partner in responsibility. Nobody can delegate away all responsibility. Only the source of the original delegated authority can release one from responsibility. Therefore, the supervisor has a relationship with the total work force under his or her jurisdiction because of responsibilities, created by the right to act, that have been delegated to the employees.

The whole concept of authority and responsibility, in fact, indicates three ways in which decisions become crucial to an effective and efficient operation. Each time one attempts to exercise authority, decisions must be made in terms of how to exercise it authoritatively or democratically, and decisions must be made with regard to the specific actions to be taken by either the supervisor or a subordinate. Each time one attempts to respond to his or her own responsibility, there is both an opportunity and a requirement to make decisions, and those decisions must be within the framework of the existing authority.

In dealing with one's subordinates, the authority–responsibility factors create an additional factor of accountability. What happens when the subordinate either cannot or will not respond to the right to act that has been delegated to him or her? This situation may, in fact, create one of the more difficult decisions that a supervisor must face. It often requires a preliminary decision about the use of established standards and the use of some mechanism to monitor the subordinate's behavior. When the monitoring process indicates that the response is either inadequate or not forthcoming, the hard decision involves how to pursue corrective action. When the supervisor fails in this key decision, it is the "cannot" and "will not" type of employee that shapes the outcome of the operation.

DECISIONS IN A DEMOCRATIC ORGANIZATION

Since the era of personhood that emerged during the 1960s with the various rights movements—civil rights, women's rights, workers' rights, patients' rights, etc.—there has emerged in health care facilities a more democratic process of operational decision making. Exhibit 3-1 portrays such an organizational format.

Since rights suggest responsibility, a recognized need for supported accountability has emerged in management systems. Basic in the principles of democratic government is the separation of the legislative, the executive, and the judicial forces. When one person or one group can legislate, execute, and judge, there is no structure for accountable behavior. One will not legislate what one cannot do. If one did legislate and did execute, one would not judge the legislation and the execution of that legislation in any way other than favorably. It is essential in government to have a democratic system of checks and balances. It is equally necessary in a democratic organizational structure within a hospital. Exhibit 3-1 demonstrates the separation of these three forces.

EXHIBIT 3-1

PARTICIPANT MANAGEMENT CHART (full scale)

ORGANIZATION	HOSPITAL SYSTEMS	HOSPITAL	DEPARTMENT	WORK UNIT	WORKER
Government	J				
Board of Trustees	E	J			
Administration	L	E	J		
Department head		L	E	J	
Supervisor			L	E	J
Worker				L	L E

J — Judicial function: the right to judge, by measurement or evaluation based on predetermined specified standards, the quality and effectiveness of both the legislation and its execution, and to take corrective action or exercise control when legislation and/or execution is inappropriate or ineffective.

E — Executive function: the right to accept or reject recommended legislation, to implement what is accepted, and to provide instruction prior to the rejection of inappropriate legislation.

L — Legislative function: the right to decide what to recommend.

Authority is not lost when one delegates to subordinates the right to legislate. It is merely the right to offer recommendations or suggestions, subject to review and acceptance or rejection by the executive. The artistic executive accepts and rewards when the legislation is good, but rejects and teaches what is wrong when the legislation is poor. Having effectively absorbed this information, the subordinates will then reject poor legislation themselves, unless they have other information that is important. In that case, the exchange of vital information often protects the supervisor from foolishly rejecting what may be appropriate recommendations or legislation.

One's superior serves in the judicial role, which is a more complex role. It requires that there be standards by which to measure, that there be knowledge of norms (created by human behavior), and that the standards be used to measure the norm. A decision or judgment whether the norm is either plus, equal, or minus the standard is then rendered. The decision prepares the way for appropriate control, which is defined here as the exercise of corrective action.

The real significance of the participative management chart (Exhibit 3-1) lies in the recognition that at each level of the organization, the legislative, executive, and judicial forces are separated. Each force provides an opportunity for the appropriate types of decisions. The subordinate decides what to recommend, but the executive decides what to accept or reject and how to implement what is accepted. Those who judge must decide on the appropriateness of both the legislation and the execution, and must further decide on what collective action needs to be implemented to maintain adequate control. The chart also shows that, at any level of the organization, one legislates for a superior, executes for one's own level of jurisdiction, and judges the actions of subordinates. Therefore, the hospital supervisor legislates (makes recommendations) regarding the operation of his or her department, subject to the review and acceptance or rejection by the department head. That same supervisor executes legislation received from the work unit but, at the same time, must establish the standard, identify the norms of what is happening, and make decisions about the adequacy of performance, exercising corrective action as needed.

THE PROCESSES OF DECISION MAKING

Since decision making is described as a process, it can be detailed in a series of sequential steps, known as a procedure. Exhibit 3-2 outlines the appropriate sequence of steps, but the supervisor is confronted with a new decision—one that has not been made before. In examining the steps, it is important both that the sequence be maintained and that all steps be achieved. A great danger is the pressure to reach a decision quickly, which often negates the validity of the decision because one or

EXHIBIT 3-2

ANTICIPATING A DECISION-MAKING PROCESS

Group or individual _____ **Date** _____

Suggested sequence: Describe briefly the situation in which there is a difference opinion or viewpoint that makes this situation an issue or a problem.

STEP 1: List the differences of opinion and the reasons they exist.

STEP 2: List the various problems reflected in this situation.

STEP 3: Select the key problem that must be resolved.

STEP 4: List the principles, concepts, theories, or known facts implicated, involved, or violated in this problem that must be considered before a decision can be determined.

STEP 5: List all possible solutions.

STEP 6: Select the single best solution and describe it fully.

STEP 7: Sequence all necessary steps that must be taken to implement this solution, determining how, when, and by whom each step should be taken.

STEP 8: Determine how, when, and by whom success or failure will be measured.

more of the steps have been overlooked. The final decision is thus handicapped.

Often a decision already made has been found from experience to be inappropriate. In this case Exhibit 3–3 outlines a somewhat detailed procedure that is intended to protect the supervisor from duplication of error or an inappropriate decision. Again, the caution is given not to change the sequence or bypass any step.

COST–BENEFIT ANALYSIS FOR DECISIONS

Health care facilities have long practiced the process of identifying expenses and then determining income. The rapid acceleration of costs in the health care delivery system has prompted government, acting under social pressure, to control the acceleration in health care costs. As a result there is a need now for cost-benefit analysis to precede decision making. Exhibit 3–4 presents the nine possible decisions that could occur, based on the combination of whether the costs increase, decrease, or stay the same, and whether the benefit or quality of the service increases, decreases, or stays the same. After each relationship of cost and benefit has been suggested, the probable decision is indicated. All supervisors, whether legislating for their superiors, executing for their work units, or judging the performance of the workers, must make decisions in the light of both costs and benefits. One should not be surprised if a decision is rejected. A good supervisor will anticipate acceptance or rejection, based on the impact of that decision on both costs and benefits.

CONCLUSION

As the management process initiates actions rather than responds to actions initiated by other sources, there is an emphasis placed on system rather than personality. This in no way diminishes the supervisor's role in the decision-making process. Through participation, the supervisor contributes to the decisions that must be made in advance to help relieve the pressure at a later time, when there may be a sense of urgency or crisis. The job descriptions and work-control program, the established personnel policies, the wage system and fringe-benefit program, and the budget system and many others simply provide a basis of information and prejudgment. These factors give the supervisor a frame of reference for guidance when a decision is needed.

All people must make simple decisions. It can be said that difficult decisions are the privilege of rank. Each one provides a unique opportunity for both personal and professional growth and development, offers an opportunity to explore various options, and requires a breadth of understanding so that the right answer can be reached. Each one enables the supervisor either to take charge or to stay in charge. Finally, each decision adds progress to programs and gives satisfaction in the fulfillment of one's responsibility. Knowing the art of making good decisions ensures quality and success.

EXHIBIT 3-3

REACTING TO A DECISION-MAKING PROCESS

Group or individual _____ **Date** _____

Suggested sequence: Describe an on-the-job situation that required an important decision. Examine this decision in terms of the following.

STEP 1: What was the problem?

STEP 2: How were you made aware of this problem?

STEP 3: What were the facts behind this problem?

STEP 4: What was the decision?

STEP 5: How did you arrive at this decision?

STEP 6: Describe the significant symptoms surrounding this problem as you saw them at that time.

STEP 7: Describe the underlying causes of this problem as you saw them at that time.

STEP 8: Were the causes of the problem within your scope of control or responsibility?

STEP 9: What were your alternative decisions?

STEP 10: What was your final decision?

STEP 11: What was the effect of your final decision as a means of resolving the problem or situation?

STEP 12: Did possible side effects either alter, affect, or influence this final decision? Describe why or why not.

STEP 13: Was this final decision, as viewed now, the best possible decision, and if not, how should it be different?

STEP 14: Who was to evaluate the success or failure of your decision?

STEP 15: How and when was the decision evaluated, and what were the results?

EXHIBIT 3-4

COST-BENEFIT ANALYSIS PROCESS FOR DECISION MAKING

The difficulty in reaching decisions at the management or administrative level can often be overcome if two separate concepts are clearly identified in any proposal that requires a decision. *Effectiveness* means doing the right job, e.g., pursuing a correct health care program in response to realistic human need. *Efficiency* means doing the job right, and relates to the appropriate utilization of resources required in the performance of the right job, including facilities, equipment, materials, and manpower, all of which can be reduced to dollars and cents (costs). By careful analysis of any proposal, its impact on the health care delivery program versus its impact on costs indicates an obvious recommended decision, as described in the chart below.

COST	BENEFIT	DECISION	DESCRIPTION
Up	Down	No	With the current emphasis on cost containment, there is certainly no justification to decide in favor of a proposal that decreases benefits while increasing costs.
Same	Down	No	Even though cost is not affected, if a proposal decreases the benefit, the obvious decision should be negative.
Down	Down	?	There are people, particularly those in government and those responsible for reimbursement of health care costs, who suggest that when cost and benefit are both reduced, the answer should probably be affirmative. There is a limit to what patients are willing to pay but, in general, there is still some degree of unwillingness to receive less even if the cost is less. Such a proposal that impacts negatively on both costs and benefits, therefore, requires detailed study, with some understanding of the impact on the recipients of such health care programs. This is a difficult decision.
Up	Same	No	There is a reluctance to pay more for the same benefit, despite the continued spiral in inflation. The high degree of sensitivity about health care ser-

Exhibit 3–4 (continued)

COST	BENEFIT	DECISION	DESCRIPTION
			vices suggests that a decision in this case be negative.
Same	Same	No	There appears to be little justification to provide a new proposal that would have no appreciable impact on benefit or cost. Why make a change that neither improves the program nor decreases costs? The suggested decision is negative.
Down	Same	Yes	The reality of cost-containment efforts can be achieved in a proposal that actually reduces costs while maintaining intact the benefits of the program. For such a proposal, the obvious decision is affirmative.
Up	Up	?	Any proposal that improves the benefits but, at the same time, increases costs requires serious study. There was a time that patients were willing to pay more provided they received more, but this is not so at present. Although one's emotions might suggest a positive decision, under present cost-containment pressure the decision is likely to be negative.
Same	Up	Yes	Obviously, if one can submit a proposal to impact positively on program improvement, upgrading benefits but without appreciably changing costs, an affirmative decision is justified.
Down	Up	Yes	The ideal proposal is one that reduces costs while it increases benefits. There is no justification for any decision other than affirmative.

marketing
of hospital
resources

(This chapter was written at the special request of the authors by Gerald W. Fuller, FHFMA, Vice President of Finance, Mid-Maine Medical Center, Waterville, Maine)

Considering the traditions and ethics of the health care industry, the question "Why market hospital resources?" is appropriate, particularly in a decentralized management-oriented facility. Most managers associate marketing with television commercials, billboards, newspapers, or radio announcements. One may also conjure up the vision of a salesman approaching someone to "close a deal" for a product or service. When we apply these thoughts to the marketing of health care services, many find the idea of marketing to be abhorrent! However, we are not advocating the marketing of appendectomies, coronary care, or similar direct services provided to patients. We are discussing expansion of the financial base of hospitals.

Some of the reasons why marketing of hospital resources is necessary are all too familiar. There are pressures to keep patient charges at the lowest possible level, pressures such as government regulation, public attitude, and the patient's ability to pay. Counterpressures that force patient charges upward are inflation, regulation, new technology, and inadequate third-party (e.g., insurance) cost reimbursement. Moreover, there certainly are limits to cost-containment efforts. The activities of various governmental review groups have also put upward pressure on patient charges. The pressures from these efforts involve decreasing the length of stay and eliminating unnecessary admissions.

The practical effect of these actions is an impact on the mix of patients and the intensity of care. As the patient mix begins to shift toward the more acutely ill with a concurrent increase in intensive care, per-diem and per-stay costs are driven upward. The pressure to provide less expensive alternatives to inpatient hospital care, such as subacute care, home care, and health maintenance organizations (HMOs), is also present. Sooner or later we will reach a crossroad where we may have to sacrifice the quality of care and reduce the quantity of services. To avoid these actions, we must devise ways to increase the volume and types of services we provide in order to spread fixed overhead more widely and thereby reduce unit costs. These reduced unit costs should have the effect of reducing patient charges, or should at least slow down the rate of increase.

Having established the need to market hospital resources, let us now look at some of the goals that should be part of a marketing program. These goals are the following.

1. Increase patient service volume.
2. Expand into providing new health care services.
3. Change behavior patterns (shift utilization patterns) among providers.
4. Develop new non-health care services related to capabilities.

With these goals in mind let's turn our attention to identification of potential areas for growth.

The first area to look at should be existing patient services (increasing patient service volume). Some of the categories ready for growth may include preadmission testing, subacute care as found in skilled nursing facilities, boarding care, intermediate care facilities, outpatient surgical units, outpatient therapy services, and home care.

Next we should look for ways to develop outside work volume for ancillary services. Some of the ways to develop this outside volume may include providing a pickup and delivery service from physicians' office buildings, providing testing services for veterinarians, and providing tests for various community-sponsored clinics dealing with venereal disease, pregnancy, family planning, hypertension screening, lead-poisoning screening, and so on.

A third area we should consider for growth is that of midwifery services and family-oriented obstetrical units.

Next we should identify potential new patient services. Most corporations and some smaller businesses have annual physical examination programs for their executives and other employees. Hospitals should seriously consider the development of a service to provide these physicals on an annual basis, which may involve contracting with various industries to run their employee health programs, including the testing of hearing for employees who work in high-noise locations.

Disease-specific screening programs for industry could be promoted, depending on the geographic area. Screening programs could be developed for lead poisoning, black-lung disease, breast cancer, diabetes, glaucoma, and so on. Another new patient service could be to advise industry, on a fee-for-service basis, on the risks they are encountering vis-à-vis the Occupational Safety and Health Administration (OSHA) requirements. Yet another possibility for new services could include subacute care and home care, if they are not already offered by the hospital.

We should also consider creating specialty clinics for the community at large. Some of these clinics could be for alcohol detoxification, alcohol rehabilitation, chronic pain, obesity, diabetes, inpatient and outpatient dentistry, and psychiatry. Does the hospital have a podiatric department? If not, is there a need for those services in the community and, if so, should the hospital provide them?

Some inpatient services to consider, if they are not already available, and that do not have a great impact on ancillary service departments, are psychiatry, physical rehabilitation, and alcohol rehabilitation. Some very sophisticated inpatient services should also be considered; these services provide a large spin-off effect on ancillary departments. Units for cancer, burns, open-heart surgery, and organ transplantation are examples.

The full use of hospital-based subspecialists is often neglected in community hospitals. The recruitment of family practitioners, endocrinologists, oncologists, neurologists, nephrologists, rheumatologists, etc., often has a very positive effect on inpatient and outpatient utilization. In addition, the referral patterns both within the medical staff and from outside the medical staff may improve as a result of the recruitment of some of these subspecialists.

Intrastaff referral patterns should be closely scrutinized. Are all your medical staff members aware of the various subspecialties that are available within the institution? One idea that has been used to improve referral patterns is the publication of a one-page biographical sketch of each medical staff member, with special emphasis on areas of expertise.

If there is an HMO in your service area, should the hospital consider associating with that HMO or some other type of prepaid service organization? If there is none available, should the hospital consider formation of its own HMO or prepaid health care plan?

Is there an adequate ambulance service in your area? If not, hospitals should seriously consider the creation of such a service.

The creation of satellite facilities, such as family-practice units, emergency first aid stations, or traveling clinics, are often viable alternatives to the creation of in-house capabilities. This action not only broadens the base of patient referrals to the hospital, but also improves the image of the hospital in the communities served.

Are some of the physicians on the staff about to retire and, if so, what is going to happen to each one's practice? Have you considered buying the practice from the physician and selling it to a newly recruited physician of the same specialty?

Is there an adequate public transportation system for prospective or existing patients in the outlying areas of your service area? If not, will the creation of a bus service help bring patients to either the hospital or some of the previously mentioned satellite facilities?

Finally, regarding new patient services, can your hospital get involved in providing services to smaller hospitals in your service area or beyond? Opportunities are often good for the creation of new patient services (or broadening the base of existing services) for other hospitals.

We will now direct our attention to several non-patient services that the hospital can provide to the community. The first possibility to explore is the selling of existing non-patient services such as those described in the following paragraphs.

Most hospitals have on their staffs very capable senior managers who would be excellent *management consultants* for other hospitals, doctors' office complexes, or service agencies within the area, such as nursing homes, YMCAs, Boys' Clubs, The Red Cross, or senior citizen housing.

Also available is a pool of *technical personnel* who could provide consulting services to various industries or agencies within the community. These services include financial planning, engineering, design, interior decorating, systems analysis, data processing, personnel administration, and so on.

Have you considered providing *food catering* to nursing homes, industries with cafeterias, schools, or social events within the community?

The *billing and collection departments* of most hospitals are usually very complex operations, and provide another fruitful opportunity to sell services. Billing and collection services could be sold to doctors, lawyers, dentists, small businesses, service agencies, and so on.

Have you considered the possibility of creating a *collection agency* for the collection of delinquent accounts? If not, you could consider the development of such an agency, whose profits could provide your hospital with a free collection service.

Those hospitals with sophisticated *data processing systems* could consider sharing time with other hospitals, or contracting with other hospitals to provide data processing services. In addition, credit unions or small banks in your area may require data processing services but cannot afford their own full-blown data processing department. How about the Health System Agency (HSA) in your area? Do they have a need for data processing services and, if so, could you provide those services?

Housekeeping also has the potential to expand the financial base of the hospital. There are many small offices and agencies within your area that could benefit from the expertise of your housekeeping department, such as doctors' offices, dentists' offices, lawyers' offices, small hospitals in the area, nursing homes, boarding homes, and so on.

How about the *maintenance department*? Does your hospital have the capability to contract grounds keeping for other institutions or businesses in your community? Some hospitals in the northern climates have their own snowplowing capabilities. These services are usually sporadic. Is it possible to contract to provide snowplowing services to some locations that do not require immediate clearance of snow? If so, can your hospital accommodate them?

The *ownership and rental* of various types of buildings within the community could well be a lucrative proposition. Is there a need for rental housing, offices, or commercial/industrial space? If so, can your hospital provide for some of these needs?

The creation of a *medical office complex* very close to the hospital can usually be made into a break-even or profit operation and, at the same time, enhance the patient flow through the hospital by having the doctors' offices very close to the institution. There are several models for creation of medical office complexes near hospitals. These models include: ownership by the hospital and rental of office space; leasing of land to other individuals for their own building; condominiums; or the sale of land for offices, nursing homes, or other health care facilities.

Is there any *excess or underutilized space* within the hospital building? If so, is it possible to rent some of the conference space to small churches in the area on Sundays and certain evenings? Is some of your underutilized space the kind that could be rented to some business?

There is normally an unmet need in most communities for *day care services.* In areas that have a heavy concentration of industry operating on a three-shift basis, there is often a need, 24 hours a day, 7 days a week, for day care centers for children or for the elderly. If the hospital has some underutilized space, could the provision of such day care services be a viable option? Day care centers for the elderly and the young also provide a convenient service for those hospital employees who need it.

Hospitals should consider the operation of either related or unrelated *businesses.* Some of these businesses include optical shops, travel agencies, tax services, answering services for physicians, bus services (as mentioned earlier), and for-profit pharmacies and gift shops.

After a hospital has identified the areas in which it wishes to expand services, create new patient services, or provide non-patient services, the next step is to identify the target population for which the services are to be provided. When trying to define the target population, remember the following points.

1. There is a different target population for each service to be considered. For example, if we are talking about expanding currently existing patient services, we must examine the need for those services, whether or not those service needs are being met in another way. If the needs are not being met, are other hospitals or health care facilities either capable, or planning to become capable, of fulfilling those particular needs?

2. The second consideration in defining the target population is to determine the primary target for the particular service being considered. Is the target your own medical staff, the medical staffs of nearby hospitals, industry, small businesses in your area, or the community in general?

3. Some of the more important targets are the following.
    a) The physicians on your own medical staff or the medical staffs of other hospitals should be taken into account. Considerations in targeting physicians include an analysis of the degree of specialization available to your hospital, as well as the age distribution of the medical staff. If the determination is made that there is not adequate medical staff available for some of the proposed new services, it will become necessary to develop

and expand recruitment efforts in order to attract physicians appropriate for the services to be provided.

b) The patient is a second important target. In this case it is extremely important to define the service area and to recognize that there is a different service area for each service being considered. Therefore, it is necessary to develop a hospital profile that indicates a service area for each existing subspecialty on the medical staff and areas for potential subspecialties. When looking at service areas, it should be determined whether or not the existing services are being utilized to the maximum degree. If not, the reasons for the underutilization should be determined, and a plan of action to correct any deficiencies should then be developed.

c) Other institutions in the service area are also important targets. The potential for the development of cooperative efforts should be considered, such as sharing of laundry facilities, materials management services, computers, and so on. Furthermore, the referral patterns of the physicians in other institutions should be studied.

d) . The fourth target to be considered relates primarily to non-patient service potential. We have mentioned previously many of the potential sources, and depending on the service being contemplated, the targets for each service may include the local HSA, the general public, doctors' offices, dentists' offices, lawyers' offices, local service agencies, other businesses in the community, and more.

Once an institution has identified both the service areas in which it wishes to expand the financial base of the institution and the target population for each service, the next step in any marketing effort is the development of criteria for determining and evaluating the feasibility of each service. Some of the considerations in the development of criteria are as follows.

1. Compatibility with the essential thrust and image of the hospital must be determined. Does the particular service relate well to the hospital mission and goals? If not, does it seem reasonable to attempt to provide the service anyway, and should the mission and goals be broadened?

2. Capacity limitations are a second consideration in determining feasibility. Concerns in analyzing the capacity limitations include demands on management capability and time, common use of resources and facility capacity in terms of space, financial resources, and personnel.

3. An attempt must be made to determine what impact any new or expanded service will have on the institution. Some facts to be considered include the following.

   a) *Physician relationships.* Does a contemplated service conflict or compete with the medical staff? If so, it may be counter-productive.

   b) *Staffing.* If new staffing is required, will it be available? Secondly, will there be any problem with any existing union?

   c) *Other institutions.* How will the other institutions respond to an aggressive marketing effort by your hospital? Will it destroy or harm any good working relationships that exist?

   d) *Community.* The attitude and receptiveness of the community on which the hospital depends for support must be assessed.

   e) *Finance.* Some questions which need to be asked in determining the feasibility of any particular project involve the return on investment, risk, a market survey (is there a need?), spin-off benefits, continuing versus one-shot improvement in the financial base, discounted cash flow studies, and tax impact (unrelated business income).

   f) *Legal considerations.* Is it legal? Will it require corporate restructuring? Will we pursue the project through litigation if necessary? Assuming that a project is legal, it may well be worth considering formation of a separate for-profit corporation for some of the activities described earlier. In this way the hospital can sell services at cost to the corporation, and the corporation can generate profits to be returned to the hospital in the form of dividends or charitable donations, the assumption being that the for-profit corporation is a wholly owned subsidiary.

   g) *Planning agency.* We must carefully consider whether planning agency approval is required for any specific projects. Will the creation of a tax service or catering service for the community be considered a new service for the hospital and, if so, will planning agency approval be required? In addition, it probably is advisable to gain the support of the HSA or other planning agencies when considering the expansion of the hospital's financial base into nontraditional types of services.

Once the feasibility of a project has been confirmed, strategies should be found for planning, developing, and implementing the service. In this regard it is extremely important to involve all the affected parties at a very early stage in the planning process. In order to rationally expand the financial base into nontraditional areas, it is important that the management of the institution be enthusiastically behind the marketing effort, or it will be doomed to failure from the very beginning.

In addition, management should gain the support of the medical staff and the Governing Board at a very early stage. After support from the management, Board, and medical staff is gained, the new services must be sold to the target population and to that portion of the institution that would be directly involved in providing the service. The targets must be analyzed to determine their relationship to other providers of similar services. An awareness of how to sell products needs to be developed, and an understanding of the criteria by which the target decides to change suppliers of particular services is necessary. In addition, it may be necessary to assign the marketing function to someone on the staff, or to create a marketing staff within the hospital.

After strategies for planning, developing, and implementing services are found, it is necessary to develop the program. Some of the considerations in program development are presented below.

When an institution is considering a financial expansion of its base by increasing current services or creating new services, one of the best methods for doing so may be to establish the hospital as a referral center using an educational thrust. For example, the development of a physician training program, management training program, medical conference, registered nurse training, industrial health team training program, OSHA training program, and certain other educational efforts may be possible.

We have already briefly discussed corporate flexibility by suggesting the formation of a wholly owned subsidiary for the for-profit activities being contemplated. Another approach could be the creation of a foundation with wholly owned, for-profit subsidiaries. An advantage to the foundation approach is that, properly structured, the activities of subsidiaries can be removed from government control. In addition, the provision of a service by a foundation's wholly owned, for-profit subsidiary reduces the probability of charges by the business community that the hospital is engaging in unfair competition. A third advantage to this approach is that turning over some of the loss leaders in the hospital to the for-profit subsidiary is possible, for example, data processing, laundry, and so on. Another advantage to this type of subsidiary is that the hospital can sell services to the corporation at cost, thereby meeting one of the goals of improving financial viability by spreading overhead and other operating costs over a broader base.

Other factors to be considered during the marketing of new or expanded services are included in the following list.

- In the development of corporate flexibility, it is essential to protect the not-for-profit status of the institution.
- Timing is very important in the development of a new service. The service must be introduced at a time when the service is needed and when the competition is most vulnerable.

- For every project, particularly non-patient services, a bail-out plan must be developed prior to implementation.
- Each service must stand on its own, and a system for precise accountability must be developed. It can then be determined whether the goals of the service are being met.
- Pricing is an important factor in the development of new services. In the development of pricing techniques, we must consider marginal cost pricing, attractive or "deal" prices, and the competitive price. In addition, volume discounts should be provided.
- The last consideration in a marketing effort should be to develop a process for an ongoing evaluation of the program. This involves keeping up with changes in the external environment, keeping in close touch with the internal environment, the maintenance of optimal relationships to capacity, and the changing delivery patterns of health care.

CONCLUSION

It is essential that hospitals develop new services, and it is also necessary that existing services be expanded. We have seen from the prior discussion that the innovative hospital has a virtually unlimited potential for expansion into new service areas.

A successful marketing effort will enhance the financial viability of the institution; it will force long-range planning by the institution; it will increase involvement and support of the medical staff and governing board for the institution; it will enhance the hospital's image and credibility; and it will enhance the training and development of the management staff.

As a final comment, I believe it is not optional but *essential* to expand the resources of the hospital through marketing in order to remain financially viable and continue the basic mission of the hospital: to provide high quality patient care at the lowest possible cost consistent with available resources.

SOURCES

"How to Expand the Hospital's Revenue Sources." Seminar conducted by the American College of Hospital Administrators, New Orleans, October 1975.

Material presented by James T. Whitman, Certified Public Accountant (CPA), FHFMA, at the Hospital Financial Management Education Foundation Annual National Institute, Boulder, Colorado, June 1977.

human resource management

It is appropriate in a discussion on decentralized hospital management that we address "human resource management." *Management* is an activity that includes setting goals, formulating plans, marshaling resources and allocating them to specific activities, organizing and directing those activities, and controlling the organization that results. *Human resources* focuses our attention on the labor component, which is of primary importance in the health care industry. In spite of the impact of technology and the importance of capital facilities and equipment, we remain a service-oriented industry that depends primarily on the input of the labor component. The health care industry employs 3,108,000 equivalent full-time personnel, "equivalent" being defined as regular full-time employees plus the figure resulting from part-time hours summed, then divided by 40. Labor costs accounted for approximately 54 percent of total hospital costs in 1976. The supervisor attempting to control cost increases or implement cost reductions in his or her department will find that personnel costs provide the greatest opportunity for success. If we are to meet the public's demand for cost containment, those of us who are responsible for managing human resources must learn to control our payroll costs. If we fail, whatever limits are achieved will be credited to outside intervention and serve as the impetus for additional bureaucratic controls. Managing human resources to contain cost increases at appropriate levels will require careful planning of services to be provided, constant reevaluation of existing services and monitoring of productivity and efficiency, imaginative and innovative use of people to keep up with advancing technology, and skillful management of people when reallocations of labor resources or reductions in force are indicated.

PLANNING FOR COST CONTAINMENT

Before planning for efficient and effective use of human resources can begin, management must have the necessary information on which to base decisions that will become the foundation for future plans. In addition to providing the basis for planning, that information becomes useful in monitoring and controlling system performance. Essential information includes the following.

1. Basic geographic and demographic characteristics of the hospital's service area
2. Broad-based epidemiological data
3. A catalogue of health services available to the service population
4. Health-service-utilization statistics for the service area
5. Comparative cost data for similar health services in different areas
6. Labor costs for each productive center or hospital service

7. Wage and salary survey data
8. Productivity data
9. Labor-turnover statistics

Items 1 through 5 are usually compiled by regional health system agencies (HSAs). Items 6 through 9 are specific to individual institutions and are the responsibility of each institution's management.

For hospitals that are already using departmental budgeting as a control technique and a supervisory development method, departmental cost data are probably already available in the financial office. Standardized cost reporting, a long-sought approach that can provide comparable cost data for all participating hospitals, will permit management to analyze labor costs more easily for similar services at several hospitals.

Wage and salary data are now commonly shared by hospital personnel administrators in periodic surveys conducted by hospital associations or other regional groups, including Chambers of Commerce. Changes in wage levels often reflect changing patterns of worker utilization or changing requirements for licensure.

Productivity data are gathered and published with comparative data by the American Hospital Association's Hospital Administrative Services (HAS). Frankly, the usefulness of the data is doubtful because of nonstandardized reporting; much additional effort is needed in this area. However, at present the HAS statistics are the most commonly used and most accessible productivity measures available to hospital supervisors. These data represent some of the basic input into the planning process and are later useful in monitoring actual system performance as compared with planned objectives. Two phenomena that have a direct impact on staffing and cost and that give rise to the need for careful planning are (1) changing patterns of utilization and (2) service changes dictated by changing technology.

Changing utilization may be attributed to demographic changes in the service area such as increasing population or changes in age distribution, or it may result from changes in the availability of competing health services. The arrival of an obstetrician on the staff of a nearby hospital will clearly have an effect on the utilization of the obstetrical service at your hospital. Therefore, the arrival should also have a direct effect on the staffing pattern you use in your facility. The departure or death of that obstetrician may have an equally important effect in the opposite direction.

In the health care field, many service changes are the direct result of changing technology. For example, the development of the techniques for hemodialysis, and the subsequent acceleration of the application of that technology resulting from changes in reimbursement methods, gave rise to an entirely new service at some medical centers and required recruitment, training, and organization of highly special-

ized staffs of technicians, nurses, and physicians. The staffing requirements have had an obvious impact on costs at those centers. Research
that suggested a correlation between mammography and subsequent
breast cancers has likewise had a drastic negative effect on the utilization of mammography, and thus has reduced demand for personnel
skilled at performing those examinations.

Hospital organizations that fail to adequately consider the effects
of various factors, including technology, on the utilization of their
services miss many opportunities to contain costs. The failure to recognize the need for new or expanded services may result in unnecessary
overtime or callback expenses, and the failure to recognize decreasing
utilization of existing services results in the lack of reallocation of
scarce resources to areas of greater need, or the lack of outright cost-
savings achievement.

It is entirely possible that establishing new services may lower
overall costs. The establishment of an intravenous administration team
may result in the savings of several staff nursing positions in various
nursing units. Therefore, it is not always the conservative approach that
results in cost savings.

Carefully monitoring utilization and thoroughly planning expansions and contractions of services is the first step in developing realistic
staffing patterns and achieving effective cost control. The result of the
planning process, like most budgeting processes, consists of a projection
of demand or utilization and a target figure for costs (in this case labor
costs) per unit of service. As usual, the projected labor costs imply projected volume of labor and cost per labor unit; here is where the wage
and salary survey data are useful. If we could all develop meaningful
comparative data and produce reasonably accurate plans, we would be
well on our way to achieving cost control.

ESTABLISHING APPROPRIATE STAFFING LEVELS
AND REEVALUATING EXISTING SERVICES

The same data used for initial planning should be used for evaluating
an organization's cost performance and for establishing or reestablishing
appropriate staffing levels. Subjective judgments will be needed as well
as objective analyses of data. If the utilization of an existing service
drops or the service operates at a level that cannot reasonably justify
the minimum level of staffing necessary to provide that service, we suggest that very careful consideration should be given to eliminating the
service if at all feasible. In these situations, cooperative services and
shared systems are very logical. Nevertheless, we recognize that in some
cases the service is justified regardless of the cost per unit, but the justification should be a conscious decision based on facts and not just
something that happens because the service is already established.

Establishing staffing levels to meet targeted costs per unit of service becomes a relatively easy process if a sufficient, stable demand is present. However, in cases of marginal utilization or extremely fluctuating demand, imagination and innovation will be required. In these cases variable staffing patterns, floating personnel, on-call labor pools, temporary service agencies, and other schemes intended to vary the level of labor input to meet service demand are useful.

Proposals for new services or expansion of existing services should be evaluated based on whether realistic estimates of demand or utilization justify the proposed staffing and whether the proposed staffing is at least the minimum required to provide the service. It may work out statistically to propose establishing an emergency service staffed with one physician, but one person cannot provide the minimum staffing level necessary to offer comprehensive emergency service. There must be a so-called "critical mass" of demand for the proposed service. Expansions of existing services can be considered in the same manner.

A more difficult question that has the attention of professional-standards-review organizations is whether the projected utilization, however feasible, is appropriate for the service population. Many observers recognize that in medical care, service creates demand. It is felt that in many cases, even though costs per unit of service are within reasonable limits, the volume of service is artificially high because of overutilization by physicians with a stake in the volume of service provided. The explosion in the number of automated laboratories illustrates the point. A computerized chemical analyzer can perform basic blood chemistry tests at a fraction of the cost of manually done tests. However, to be cost-effective, a very high volume of tests must necessarily be performed. Hence the "laboratory profile" has become the pattern. The physician can have a series of twelve chemical tests done at a cost of, say, one dollar per test. Obviously that is more desirable than having one test performed manually at a cost of, say, six dollars. Or is it desirable, when you realize that the total cost is twelve rather than six dollars? This question, though important, is not within our sphere of concern here. The primary concern for the institutional manager is whether the cost per unit of service is appropriate.

ANALYZING PRODUCTIVITY

The question to be answered now is, "What is the appropriate cost per unit of service?" As we indicated earlier, cost has two components: (1) cost per unit; and (2) volume. The cost per hour of labor can readily be determined by the use of wage and salary surveys. The individual hospital has little control over labor cost per hour except on a very short-term basis. If a hospital fails to remain competitive because it pays low wages or benefits, it will lose the qualified staff it has and will be unable to recruit equally qualified personnel. The situation to be avoided is that of paying more than is necessary by permitting extravagant pay increases for tenure or by employing overqualified personnel. Labor costs can often be reduced by using lower-skilled persons to perform only lower-skill tasks as well as using higher-skilled personnel to the maximum by restricting them to higher-skill tasks. Substituting a lower-paid employee for a higher-paid employee is an obvious route to cost reduction.

The volume statistic, workhours per unit of service, is the critical one when reviewing labor costs. It is for this statistic that productivity or efficiency indexes have been developed, and it is usually by affecting this statistic that management engineers earn their salaries. Productivity indexes are merely guidelines, developed with experience in determining how much labor of a specific type is required to do a specific task. A second step in calculating the volume statistic is a careful determination, by either work sampling or job analysis, how many times the specific task is actually performed in a given institution. One then predicts, by analysis of past experience, when the performance of that task will be required. Time study and regression analysis are tools of the management engineer.

A favorable effect on the cost-per-unit-of-service statistic can be achieved in one of three ways: (1) decrease the labor cost per hour; (2) decrease the number of labor hours used; or (3) increase the units of service output. Cost containment can be achieved by cost reduction either in an absolute sense or by realizing a greater output for the same expense.

KEEPING PACE WITH TECHNOLOGY

One trend in modern medicine that leads to dramatic cost increases is technological advance and the resulting specialization of labor. The technology explosion in hospitals is so obvious that it hardly requires examples. More important to this discussion is the accompanying trend towards specialization of personnel. Specialization leads to higher cost per hour and less flexibility in assigning people with special skills to perform a variety of unspecialized tasks. The undesirable cost consequences are most obvious in two areas: (1) clinical laboratories and (2) respiratory therapy departments. Managers must be careful to avoid employing and paying people on the basis of credentials rather than on the basis of the tasks actually required to be performed. Managers should also exert maximum influence to fully use necessary people with special skills to perform nonspecialized tasks during slack times. The pitfall to be avoided, however, is unnecessarily hiring skilled persons to do unskilled tasks.

Technological advance can be used to advantage when it permits the replacement of labor with less expensive capital input. However, experience leads us to believe that replacing people with machines is often planned and seldom achieved. Most hospital laboratories represent the worst example of the expense of advancing technology.

ACHIEVING LABOR COST REDUCTION

If we do our jobs well, we will be able to identify areas in which changing technology and changing utilization give us the opportunity to reduce costs by reducing labor input. In some areas we can actually reduce the staff. The problem becomes one of dealing compassionately with people. In most cases we will want to avoid layoffs because hospitals are proud of their record of providing secure employment. One way to achieve labor reductions is by the constructive use of employee turnover. A second alternative is to offer voluntary workweek reductions. Since many hospital employees are working parents or have spouses who also work, voluntary reductions in the number of regularly scheduled hours of work are often welcome. This is especially true if the hospital provides equal or nearly equal benefits for part-time and full-time employees. Having a large number of part-time workers entails some additional expense, but it also can provide desirable flexibility in staffing, resulting in long-term cost savings.

Some people advocate achieving cost reduction by making full use of employees hired under government grants and retraining programs for the unemployed. In cases where the position already exists and has been otherwise justified, this approach is definitely a useful one. However, experience also tells us to be extremely cautious about employing people with so-called "soft money." Our caution is based on a twofold concern. Firstly, the availability of government or foundation reimbursement is often used to help justify a new position that could not otherwise be justified. Secondly, the term of the soft-money program is almost always limited, and at the end of the "temporary" period, the hospital ends up with another person on the payroll in a now-established position requiring hard dollars. Using soft money is fine if it is strictly controlled; otherwise, it becomes another factor contributing to cost increases.

SUMMARY

Cost containment is possible through proper management of human resources. It requires:

- thorough planning;
- establishing appropriate staff levels;
- reevaluating existing services;
- analyzing productivity;
- keeping pace with technological change; and
- achieving cost reductions where feasible.

6

payroll
costs

A knowledge of wage and salary administration as well as other sound business practices becomes very necessary in a decentrally managed organization. Proper administration of a wage and salary program can have a profound effect on both management and employees. It can save your institution the cost caused by high turnover while attracting, retaining, and motivating capable and productive employees.

DEVELOPING A WAGE/SALARY POLICY

Before exploring the development and implementation of formal procedures and the possible utilization of varied techniques for compensating employees, a health care institution should examine the basic philosophy behind its payment of wages and salaries. This is usually summarized in an all-inclusive policy that sets the tone for other wage and salary policies. It is characterized by many variables within a particular institution. Factors determining policy are: the management's attitude toward paying prevailing rates in a community; an institution's ability to pay, influenced by its productivity and managerial efficiency; and the presence or absence of labor unions. A typical policy might read:

> Hospital X's policy is to pay fair and reasonable salaries that will (1) allow for the recruitment, retention, and motivation of capable personnel; (2) maintain internal equity, allowing employees to be rewarded on the basis of their performance and professional capabilities; and (3) further the objectives of the institution.

To meet its basic obligation to employees, the management must compensate them equitably for their contributions. To ensure this compensation, there are several fundamental requirements that must be met other than just a strict adherence to the legal requirements of both state and federal governments. The management must ensure an equitable internal wage and salary structure. The implication is that the duties and responsibilities of each job within a hospital are correctly compared with the others and that employees are paid accordingly. An equitable external structure must also be ensured, which means that compensation should be competitive with the pay for similar jobs in other hospitals in the same geographic area. Equally as important is a wage and salary structure constructed in a manner that provides incentive for employees. If a compensation program is built around these key ingredients, the needs of employees and management will be met.

It should be evident by now that the installation or maintenance of a proper wage and salary program within a health care institution is based on a number of different factors. The proper interpretation of these factors cannot be classified as an exacting science, since it involves the use of human judgment.

WAGE AND SALARY POLICIES

With some understanding of the fundamental elements of a sound wage and salary program, appropriate policies can and should be developed and implemented within your institution. These guiding principles are established by the people in top management, reflecting their business philosophies and creating the climate for all compensation actions. These managerial philosophies should influence all personnel policies, wage and salary being an integral part of the whole picture. There are many areas of integration. Hiring success, for example, depends on the ability to offer competitive wages in the recruitment of new personnel. The capacity to retain a work force and maintain a high level of morale, as well as to provide incentive for promotions, is also an area somewhat influenced by the maintenance of an adequate level of compensation. It would be misleading to indicate that proper pay policies are the sole influence in any or all employment considerations. Personnel management is a complex subject with many interlacing forces, since it deals mainly with human nature and its relationships.

Poor morale, even chaos, could prevail without established organization policies; this point is true for both small and large hospitals. Lack of consistency in the treatment of employees is probably the biggest problem area. For example, a person who aggressively complains about his salary may get larger increases than an employee who may be a high producer but is less vocal about his income. A lack of proper guidelines could play havoc with one of an institution's largest items of cost—compensation. Improper administration of salary increases could result in a large turnover rate, causing labor costs to spiral upward because of the expense of recruiting and training workforce replacements.

The written policies should be part of a formal program that includes the establishment of wage and salary ranges from a job evaluation plan. The publication and distribution of this information gives supervisors a framework for decision making, thus allowing the planning of promotions, the fair compensation of employees for their contributions to the institution, and the budgeting of employee costs. It also lessens the possibility of misinterpretation of policies, especially if they are written in a clear and concise manner.

Wage and salary policies should be written so that they are flexible enough to allow exceptions or slight deviations from the norm when necessary. Policies should never be considered static, because conditions do change both inside and outside the institution. In order to keep the policies current, some type of periodic review should be established.

A number of specific concerns should be examined after the establishment of a philosophy on wage policy.

1. *Develop a policy statement to determine base pay (minimum wage) and spell out the criteria by which it is determined*; include the legal minimum wage, minimum wage plus a percentage, a union contract, major areas of competition, and so on.

2. Based on a job evaluation or classification system, establish a base rate for each pay grade and determine by policy the number and amount of employees within each increment from minimum to maximum, including the frequency at which adjustments can be expected.

3. Consider specific policy statements on additional wage concerns, including overtime pay, call pay, report pay, shift differential pay, and so on.

4. Using policy statements, provide the means by which wages can be adjusted to accommodate factors such as temporary assignment to a higher position.

5. Using policy statements, provide the means by which the wage system itself will be accelerated to keep pace with either the cost of living or competitive wages elsewhere.

6. Establish a system of performance appraisal to ensure that the increasing value of performance is within the appropriate range to justify the increasing value of wages. Other controls may need to be established in terms of defining wage increases for tenure, wage increases for merit, and eventually wage increases for longevity.

7. In recognition of the fact that a hospital recruits through its wage program but retains through its fringe benefit program, a careful analysis should be undertaken to determine whether the basic personnel problem is one of recruitment or retention. This analysis will assist in determining whether additional money should be more appropriately placed in the wage package or in the fringe benefit package.

Just as the hospital undergoing careful budgeting has to understand and predict future costs and must thereby have an understanding of future income, so also has the employee reached a point where, in planning for personal and family requirements, he or she must be able to accurately anticipate expected income—both cash and fringe benefits. The constant pressure for added dollars should be viewed as a constant factor in wage planning. The inflationary trend in the cost of living will require more dollars to maintain the integrity of each employee's economic status.

All of the foregoing suggests not cost controls or containment, but rather the escalation of costs. We are attempting to point out that it is now necessary for health care institutions to start planning for the future. Develop sound policies on wage and salary administration. Do some wage planning. Know where you are going. Develop a program that the institution can live with, particularly regarding the payment of fair and equitable wages.

ESSENTIAL FACTS ABOUT WAGE DETERMINATION

Unless and until hospitals recognize some essential facts relative to the determination of a wage and salary program, the hospital's future wage program may be as rocky and unstable as it has been in the past. There are some facts which can be accepted as principle, since they appear to be unchanging and thus establish a solid foundation for the determination of a wage and salary system. Some of these facts are as follows.

1. Wages should purchase performance rather than buy time or talent In the historical development of wage planning in this country as reflected in the minimum wage laws, money is equated to time. For example, the minimum wage will soon be $3.35 per hour (effective January 1, 1981). This time concept reflects nothing about what an employee may or may not do in that hour. Hospitals have traditionally followed this approach. There is also a second influence that comes from certain educational institutions (those connected with hospitals through clinical education), dictating a specific rate of pay based on the academic achievement or particular talents of the worker. Thus a B.S.N. degree registered nurse (R.N.) would receive a higher rate of pay than a non-R.N. diploma graduate but a lower rate of pay than an M.S.N. degree R.N., even though all three may do the same assignments in the same way with the same degree of responsibility.

It is hoped that differing talent can lead to differing tasks and eventually to jobs with differing wages, but this certainly has not always been the case. Business and industry, using one system, have for many years concentrated on the concept of performance or productivity as the basis for wage payments. This concept has led to incentive systems and piecework systems based solely on the rate of performance. In contrast, hospitals have employed the underexperienced, the elderly, the unemployed, and in many instances those unemployable elsewhere, allowing them to function without performance standards or systems of evaluating effectiveness. What is needed is the attitude that a given wage buys performance; not time, but talent with appropriate performance requirements. Hospital management should be assured that value is received for the payroll dollars paid.

2. A wage should be an investment, not a cost or an expense As indicated above, due to the failure to purchase performance with payroll dollars, wages have actually become a cost item to the hospital. The investment of a higher wage per hour in exchange for a far better rate of performance in the same time period would actually result in a greater return for the hospital payroll dollar. Wages should, therefore, become an investment.

3. Wages respond to the supply and demand factor of economics Although hospitals would like to avoid the concept, there always exists the supply versus demand factor that pressures the hospital into paying more or that pressures the recruit into accepting less. Even so-called "objective" systems of wage determination take into account some factor based on supply and demand.

4. Management essentially controls the work to be performed but does not control the price paid to the worker Because of the influences given in the preceding paragraphs, the recognition of the supply and demand factors may well determine the wage price. The management can offer that price to attract labor, thus paying more for an unchanging performance level and increasing cost of operations. However, the management can attempt to redesign the work in such a way as to increase its net worth to the institution, thereby justifying a higher rate of pay and perhaps recruiting a more capable worker. There is still some spirit of professionalism, dedication, and service to humanity that persuades some individuals to work within a hospital system. This spirit has been diminishing over the past two decades and perhaps will continue to diminish, despite the new surge of interest in a Christian conscience and some form of Christian witness among the younger generation. It seems that hospitals will need to pay the "going rate" for labor or do without. *To merely respond with extra dollars will increase costs. To respond with work improvement to justify increased dollars can at least maintain economic stability for the institution.*

5. There is no concept of wage that is either absolute or right The question is often raised about what is the right wage to pay a particular occupation or group of workers. At best, wages are a relative value, not an absolute value. A correct wage is one that justly compensates the employee for the rate of performance rendered to the employer. If this principle were fully applied in hospitals, many employees might experience drastic wage reductions. Until we socially and legally accept the principle that each person has a right to whatever is needed to maintain his or her standard of living, there will remain the belief that the employee is expected to perform at a level that, from wages, will determine that employee's standard of living. If you want more, it has always been expected that you should do more. However, in today's society an increasingly common attitude is that if you want more, go out and demand more.

6. **Wages must be correct in their relationship not only within the institution but also between the institution and outside sources of competitive employment**   There is constant pressure both to maintain traditional patterns of relationships in wages within the hospital as well as to break such relationships. For example, the licensed practical nurse (L.P.N.) has traditionally earned three-quarters the rate of pay of the R.N. There is no absolute right or wrong in this situation. When the certified laboratory assistant was introduced into the clinical laboratory, it was determined that this individual would earn three-quarters the rate of the American Society of Clinical Pathologists (ASCP) medical technologist. In addition, as more sophisticated systems were applied to wage determinations, it was usually found that the X-ray technologist was several pay grades under the professional nurse, and the medical technologist was one pay grade under, or the same as, the professional nurse in a 15- to 18-pay-grade system. Again, there is no absolute right or wrong in this situation. However, through the years pressure by the lower-pay group to break this traditional relationship was yielded to only to result in counterpressures from the higher-pay group to again achieve the nonequity of a wage difference. As long as opinions and attitudes support such pressures rather than a system of relative values or some other organized method of value determination, they will continue to be applied.

It appears that there will be continuous difficulty in maintaining both internal and external relationships of wages on traditional grounds. Consequently, hospitals will in time be required to develop a systematic approach to relative value analysis by which wages can be determined independent of opinion, attitude, pressure, and even supply and demand to some extent.

7. **Fringe benefits are classified as collateral wages and must be as specifically defined as dollars and cents per hour, or preferably, dollars and cents per unit of production**   Although the fringe benefit has long been acknowledged as a factor in compensation that has its own unique purpose and value, the "Little Steel Formula" developed under the wage and price control systems during World War II (the Emergency Price Control Act of 1942) officially recognized fringe benefits as an indirect method of wage payment. Court decisions since that major decision have classified fringe benefits as collateral wages. Union contracts and personnel policies now require that the fringe benefits be specifically defined as dollars and cents per hour or unit of production.

8. **Recruitment is based on money—retention is based on fringe benefits**   Recruitment and retention do not always involve simply attempting to keep pace with competition in terms of both base rates and fringe benefits. It is often important to study whether recruitment —the ability to recruit qualified applicants to fill pending positions—or retention of incumbent workers is a more vital concern. Money is essen-

tially the primary recruiter. Young applicants do not seek employment because of the retirement program, the life insurance program, or the health insurance program. For the employee already on board and functioning effectively, the fringe benefits added to the wages become the essential element in retention (along with other intangible benefits such as the relationship with supervisors, the opportunity for participation and decision making, a sense of belonging, and so on).

9. Wages have a low priority when the basic wage is adequate Managers believe much too often that wages are the most important element in the employees' demand package. Actually, many people work within the hospital for reasons other than economic return, even when wages are important or even essential to the employee. It has been found in relative-value studies that when the basic wage is adequate to meet normal, expected standard-of-living requirements, wages take a low priority and often become less important to the employee than job security, the opportunity for advancement, meaningful supervisory-employee relations, a sense of personal worth, recognition and appreciation as an individual, status derived from positions of importance, influence or power, and so on. The management often gives greater emphasis to wages than do employees. To some extent, it is easier to try to buy employee satisfaction through a simple exchange of money for performance than it is to earn employee satisfaction with the less tangible working conditions.

10. The complexity of wage and salary administration requires a formal system If people will buy a system, they will usually buy what comes out of that system. It has become so difficult to attempt to justify each individual's rate of pay and pay adjustments that administrators are turning somewhat desperately toward recognition of the need for a wage and salary system. This system requires some means of job classification, the establishment of pay grades, the determination of wage ranges with minimums and maximums, an orderly system of wage increases with prescheduled dates and amounts, and periodic adjustments to recognize changes in the cost of living, merit, the labor market, productivity, longevity, or seniority. In addition, special determinations concerning differential pay, report pay, call pay, etc., must be made. Although conditions dealing with report or call pay have been established in the Fair Labor Standards Act, the law merely establishes minimum guidelines that must be equitably applied to the total hospital system.

None of these concepts are simple to fathom and accept equitably into a total system, but the effort must be made.

SUMMARY

The problems are many and the solutions are difficult, but solutions must be found and implemented if administrators are to provide a wage and salary program equitable to the employee, the patient, the public, and the institution. The problems must first be clearly defined and understood, and then the solutions must be sought to resolve each problem. Each hospital is unique. The workers in one hospital do not do exactly the same work at the same performance level as workers at a similar level in the next hospital. Even within a group of workers in the same hospital there will be differing tasks and performance rates. Therefore, it is important that administrators not duplicate the mistakes of another institution but rather attempt to be creative and to design a wage and salary program tailored to fit the needs of all concerned. A program cannot be all things to all groups, but it can create order from chaos, a system from individual pieces, and fairness from inequity. The wage and salary program of the hospital must not be a display of charity, but rather a display of justice.

Paying employees for the work they do appears to most inexperienced supervisors as a relatively easy economic exchange, i.e., a fair wage for a fair day's work. The more experienced supervisors and wage and salary analysts agree totally with the old cliché defining wage and salary administration as an art. It is the art of distributing dissatisfaction equally among all employees.

labor
turnover

The term labor turnover is an adaptation from the field of merchandising. It is defined as the gross movement of people *into* and *out of* active employment status. The index of this movement is the measurement of labor turnover, known as the "turnover rate."

Turnover is a hidden cost factor in the operation of an institution, particularly when one considers the results of an in-depth analysis completed at one large midwestern hospital. Researchers discovered that the hospital's turnover rate was 57 percent a year and that the average cost per employee was over $600. That added up to over $1 million a year, or about 2 percent of the hospital's operating budget.

Of all the complexities in supervisory management, the one pertaining to causes of labor turnover is one of the most perplexing and controversial. Although few supervisors agree on its causes or accept responsibility for controlling turnover, many who have been surveyed agreed that it is indeed costly. Thus it is not only worthy of consideration as an element of cost containment, but also, if it is controlled, turnover can contribute to a more effective and efficient department.

Fortunately, turnover can be measured. As a matter of fact, it is one of the few readily measurable aspects of the health care field's operation that can be accurately measured. Methods of measurement vary from one institution to another, depending on what each institution wants to measure. Some hospitals eliminate from consideration such items as unavoidable separations or terminations caused by illness, death, military service, moving from the area, following the spouse who transfers, and the like. Many hospitals do not include part-time or temporary workers. Others exclude losses due to pregnancies and retirement. Hospitals that ignore all these categories are basically measuring only a "quit rate." Many institutions consider the "quit rate" group as the only group over which they have some form of management control. For most purposes, this theory is probably correct. However, for cost-containment purposes one needs to look at the whole picture in order to realize any savings or cost avoidance related to attritions. Most management consultants agree that when you define "turnover," it must include retirements, discharges, deaths, resignations (adequate notice given), disabilities, part-time work, and separations caused by illness, military service, transfers, pregnancies, and quits (inadequate or no notice given). The consultants also agree that it *does not* or *should not* include temporary employees and employees acquired as a result of grants or public-service employment contracts. Once it has been agreed or determined what is to be measured, one is ready to set up a turnover equation. This is accomplished by the following sequence.

a) Determine the period to be measured (e.g., a month, a year, etc.).
b) Determine the average number of employees in the institution (or

department) by adding the number on the payroll on the first and last days of the period and then dividing this total by 2.

c) Set up the equation as follows.

$$\frac{\text{Number of terminations in given period}}{\text{Average number of employees}} \times 100 = \text{Turnover rate (\%)}$$

Annual labor turnover rates are usually computed by totaling the twelve monthly rates. For cost-containment purposes a more meaningful annual rate is the average of the twelve monthly rates. Under current state government reporting practices, most employers provide data on their employment in the pay period that includes the twelfth calendar day of the month. This figure, which approximates the mid-month total, is normally used as the base figure in computing turnover rates. Plotted on a graph, the monthly or yearly high and low figures are easily recognized, and trends from one period to another can be charted and analyzed. Measurement and analysis of turnover seeks to find out when, where, and why turnover occurs in terms of any classification that will help in explaining it. Turnover can be measured by the type of employee, including job, age, marital status, and education level, the type of job, or any other criteria that may be meaningful. Hospitals that have been successful in meeting problems of excessive labor turnover have been those that kept records and measured their turnover on at least a monthly basis.

Many hospital supervisors contend that high turnover rates in the health care field are unavoidable because the health care field is a "female-intensive" industry. However, a private study conducted among 65 large chemical and pharmaceutical laboratories revealed only moderate differences in the labor turnover of men and women chemists when they were grouped by type of degree required for the grade of work performed. Moreover, other surveys conducted in other female-intensive industries reveal that women workers have favorable records of attendance and labor turnover when compared to records of men employed at similar job levels and under similar circumstances. The favorable findings for women workers negate the necessity of measuring turnover by sex.

To be of value in the analysis of the problem, turnover figures should be available for each department of the hospital. Sometimes a relatively small group of jobs, a department, or a single type of worker is responsible for most of the turnover in the entire hospital.

The knowledge of turnover rates may not be enough to stimulate some supervisors to take a look at turnover as a means of cost containment for their departments. While personnel programs and administrative costs vary among hospitals, turnover costs can be determined by estimating the cost of each of the applicable expense items listed below. The following table lists the actual labor turnover costs for a 100- to 300-bed, nongovernment, acute care hospital in the Northeast.

Cost factors	Average cost per new employee
Recruiting (ads and trips)	$ 41.55
Hiring (interviews, medical exams)	110.00
Orientation and training (nonproductive time)	368.00
Administrative costs (booklets, forms, photos, supplies, clerical time)	8.61
Overtime (OT) resulting from unfilled personnel requisitions	27.00
Unemployment compensation	146.84
Total turnover cost per employee	$702.00

Measuring turnover and computing the cost on a regular basis is not without value. Such statistics, when properly documented and shared with those who have a responsibility to control turnover, can be very useful in effecting cost reduction.

At this point, one needs to acknowledge that some turnover is inevitable. As a matter of fact, some turnover is desirable, and a somewhat larger amount of turnover is not unhealthy. The advantages of some turnover are as follows.

- New employees can and do bring new ideas and suggestions into an organization.
- It prevents the institution from "tenure stagnation."
- It affords the department head or the administrator a good opportunity to analyze his or her labor complement.
- It can be the major element in a discreet austerity program to reduce operating costs.
- It affords others within the institution an opportunity for promotion.
- It can frequently be an avenue for the relief of troublesome individuals.

MAKING ATTRITION WORK FOR YOU

Traditionally, hospitals resolve a majority of their workflow bottlenecks, staffing and census problems, and other workforce and work distribution imbalances by pumping more people into what is frequently an already overstaffed system without the benefit of any critical analysis or justification. This method, although being an easy way of acknowledging staffing difficulties, is in reality an appeasement style of workforce planning that is being challenged and reversed as more and more pressure is being brought to bear on the health care system to contain costs. Turnover per se can be a vehicle to assist hospitals in checking escalating employee-per-bed ratios as well as affording supervisors an opportunity to selectively decide where in the department available labor dollars (freed up as a result of attrition) should be either expended or removed from the operating budget.

Either of the following two basic methods can make attrition work for you.

REPLACEMENT ANALYSIS

A coordinated analysis must be conducted to ensure that the vacated position needs to be refilled. In recognition of the cost challenge to hospitals with regard to their operating costs and the quality of services rendered, the process of replacement analysis as a basis for decision making is becoming more significant today than it was previously. The move from automatically and subjectively replacing all employees who leave the department to well-documented objective justification for a replacement is providing supervisors with the opportunity to become more aware of costs (or services rendered). With such information, the administrator can make a more realistic decision to either (1) approve plans for a replacement, (2) modify the skill requirements of the person to be recruited, (3) reject the replacement requisition, or (4) suggest to the department head certain work improvement methods for his or her department.

ATTRITION WORK-DISTRIBUTION ANALYSIS

Not until hospital supervisors have an interest and are involved in controlling work and work processes will there be an opportunity to truly bring the cost of hospital operations under control. Therefore, it is important that hospital department heads be encouraged to master some of the techniques of work simplification and work distribution. Many hospitals have chosen to contract with a variety of industrial engineers to design or investigate techniques in the institutions aimed at achieving work simplification. On occasion some economy is realized, but too often it is short-lived, and in the absence of true understanding and involvement of department heads it cannot be sustained. In contrast, there are hospitals that have chosen an in-house approach to work distribution by training supervisors in the actual techniques of simplifying work, particularly when positions in their departments are vacated. These programs have not only sustained themselves but have created within the departments a degree of curiosity and satisfaction that motivates further application of the techniques for an ongoing or continuing program of work distribution and work simplification.

The in-house approach need not be a complicated technical web of time and motion studies. One can merely identify and prudently analyze several key concerns that may indicate where the greatest value can be gained from the decision to replace or not replace a departing employee. The program will then start to bring some benefit to the institution. It is not the purpose of an in-house attrition work-distribution analysis to make industrial engineers out of hospital supervisors. However, experience has demonstrated that most supervisors have the capability to learn how to effectively analyze, improve, and implement changes in at least some of the following areas, provided that the program is a required one, endorsed and sustained by the administrator.

- Tasks that have excessive cost
- Tasks that create bottlenecks
- Tasks that are not achieving their purpose
- Tasks that are consistently performed below existing performance standards
- Tasks that create interdepartmental problems or that are shown to be unnecessary or ineffective

COST AVOIDANCES IN THE SELECTION AND PLACEMENT PROCESS

So far, we have discussed (1) how to measure turnover, (2) the cost of turnover, and (3) the methods of making attrition work for you. At this point, on the premise that a replacement must be hired, one should explore the possibility of cost avoidances.

Inadequate selection and placement methods cause an increase in the turnover rate that, in turn, becomes a hidden cost to the hospital. Fitting the right worker into a position should not be considered a simple process. Guesswork, special inspiration, or a good hunch will not assure the success of a proper worker–position match. Selecting the right worker out of a group of applicants requires the interplay of many recognized personnel techniques. It is essential that at least one of the selection processes be based on the premise of full information and disclosure of the job or position, including information seeking to gain full information about the applicant.

One of the most common selection and placement errors made by interviewers is that of painting too many rosy pictures in order to attract an ideal candidate. It is essential that honesty prevail; the interviewer should candidly point out task by task what is done, how it is done, why it is done, and how often. If there are certain unpleasant aspects of the job, the candidate should be advised of them. Improper selection of a candidate and lack of honesty in describing a job or position leads to a host of costly personnel problems. Training needs, labor turnover, grievances, poor morale, work errors, etc., can be greatly reduced if not virtually eliminated by honestly depicting the job or position.

Reflect, just for a moment, what took place the last time you hired a new employee. We may repeat the process many times each week in each month; because of constant repetition, this all-important hiring procedure becomes routine. However, since it is a new or infrequent experience to most applicants, the hiring process is not routine. What usually happens to the newly hired employee is that we give the date and time to come to work, the name of the supervisor, an explanation of the operations and location of the department to which he or she will report, how to enter the hospital, and where to record the hours worked. We probably give the employee a physical, a locker number, the rate of pay, what day is payday, and when and how much to expect for the first wage increase. We issue instructions for the kind of uniform to bring, where to change, where to eat lunch, and we may further confuse the picture by explaining how the shift rotates in regard to hours and days off. It is really no surprise that every so often, after having gone through this process, a new employee fails to appear at the right place or frequently fails to appear at all. Or, the employee starts work, works a day or two, and does not return. Because of the cost and time involved in the selection and placement process, it is imperative that all institutions conduct a formal orientation program. Each orientation session must be aimed at introducing the new employee to the people, facilities, equipment, organization, philosophies, and policies of the institution and to the new employee's specific department or work area. To be effective from a cost-containment point of view, orientation should be a concise, well-planned program held on a weekly basis.

In summary, excess expenditures of time and dollars in the selection and placement process can be avoided if hospitals carefully structure their selections and placements and avoid (1) hasty selections, (2) lack of honesty in depicting jobs or positions, and (3) hasty placements and poor orientation plans. If a job is essential and the worker selected to do that job is the right one, it is very important to get that worker off to a good start.

An employee and his or her job may be "separated" either by an action of the employer (such as discharge or retirement) or by an action of the worker (such as a quit or resignation). In hospitals, the number of discharges are insignificant. From 75 percent to 95 percent of all terminations are determined by the employee who has decided to leave, i.e., 90 percent of the time there is nothing the employer can do to preclude these employee-caused terminations and 10 percent of the time the resignations are within the control of management and can be avoided if properly handled.

BENEFITS OF AN EXIT INTERVIEW PROGRAM

It is important to know the facts behind an employee's resignation and not merely accept the simple statement the employee may give as a reason for leaving. It is also important for the administrator to know what the employee thinks of the hospital as an employer and as a place to work. A properly conducted exit interview is one way to find out.

Some hospitals have a practice of sending questionnaires to former employees one month or so after they have left the institution. Hospitals that use this procedure feel that the mail questionnaire after the fact of termination brings forth more honest comments than the face-to-face exit interview conducted on the last day of work, when the employee may be either emotional about leaving the job that he or she has been happy doing or reluctant to give the real reason for leaving if the employee is unhappy about being separated. Frequently the information gathered by mail inquiry, while providing interesting reading, is not worth the effort it costs. The most effective exit interview program is the type that gathers the information prior to the employee's leaving and on a face-to-face, one-to-one basis. Exit interviews are of great value in the identification and improvement of the following items.

1. Working conditions for other employees
2. Morale
3. Work simplification methods
4. Areas that are overstaffed or understaffed
5. Underutilization of staff

To be effective, facts gained from exit interviews must be compiled, evaluated, interpreted, classified, and passed on to the administrator. To realize cost savings, data pertaining to departments must be routed by the administrator to each department head. Included with these data should be cumulative information and suggestions that the department head can use to resolve current personnel problems, reduce labor turnover, eliminate areas of employee grievances, institute work-improvement methods, and review suggestions relative to areas of over-staffing or underutilization of staff. There should be a written follow-up report submitted by the department head indicating positive actions taken.

The following is a guide for planning and conducting an effective cost-containment exit interview program.

GUIDE FOR PLANNING AND CONDUCTING A COST-CONTAINMENT EXIT INTERVIEW PROGRAM

1. Set the time and place for the interview as soon as possible after the employee has submitted a letter of resignation. Provide comfort, convenience, and privacy.

2. Select an interviewer who is mature, sympathetic, and understanding, who has respect for the employees, and who is not considered too management-minded.

3. Assure the interviewee of privacy and that the information given will be used prudently, and explain the purpose of the program, i.e., cost containment as well as possible improvements for the benefit of the remaining employees, those to follow, and the interviewee, should he or she want to stay or return someday.

4. Conduct the interview without using leading questions or questions that can be answered with a "yes" or "no." Use questions such as, "Do you feel . . . ?", "Why do you believe . . . ?", "How does this . . . ?", "In your opinion . . . ?", and so on.

5. Pursue several areas of thought including the following points.

   a) Selection, placement, orientation
      i) Was the applicant properly qualified for the work?
      ii) Was the work correctly presented?
      iii) Was a proper introduction given to the department, the work, fellow workers, the work environment, and work relationships?
      iv) Were rules, policies, and procedures explained?
      v) Was a proper understanding of the work of the hospital, the hours of work, and the relationship of the work to patient care given?
   b) The work environment, department supervison
      i) Did the employee receive adequate and considerate supervision?
      ii) What changes are recommended in the work, duties, methods, qualifications, etc., before a replacement is employed?
      iii) What are the suggestions for improving the job?
   c) Employee needs
      i) Did the position offer security?
      ii) Was there a feeling of opportunity present in this position?
      iii) Was the work personally satisfying?
      iv) Was it the type of work in which a person could build an interest?

     v) Did the employee look forward to his or her work each day?

    vi) Was there harmony and contentment in the department?

   vii) Were all matters of pay properly and promptly answered?

  viii) What is the employee's attitude toward vacations, holiday, sick leave, insurance programs, and other benefits?

d) Views on working conditions

     i) Was the work area clean, comfortable, safe, and pleasant?

    ii) Were working hours properly explained, assigned, scheduled, and distributed?

   iii) Were grievances accepted without prejudice and acted on promptly?

   iv) Were patients and visitors treated with courtesy and compassion?

    v) Was discipline properly carried out in the department when necessary?

   vi) Were there any bottlenecks related to the job?

  vii) What tasks being performed could be eliminated or streamlined?

Basically, supervisors must exhibit interest and exercise some control over labor turnover programs before the programs can realize cost-containment benefits. Labor turnover as related to effective cost containment must be viewed as more than just employees leaving their place of employment. Labor turnover programs, as we have discussed, are not so much a set of *do's* and *don'ts* as they are a set of tools and techniques that need to be used, with corrective actions taken when necessary. Preventive labor turnover programs need to be result-oriented and expressed by some kind of remedial effort. If substandard employees have already been hired, changes need to be made in the selection process that will preclude or minimize the recurrence of this problem.

Remember, the employment of workers begins with the act of recruiting. Recruitment cost and related costs absorb a significant portion of administrative budget dollars.

8

employee
and labor
relations

Being an efficient and effective supervisor took on added complexity following the "health care amendments" (1974) to the National Labor Relations Act (NLRA), which consists of the Wagner Act (1935) and the Taft-Hartley Act (1947). These amendments extended to nearly two million nongovernment, not-for-profit, health care employees the right to unionize—"the right to engage in concerted activity for collective bargaining and other mutual aid or protection."

Facing this new dimension of supervision requires the supervisor to become familiar with the basics of the NLRA. But the efficient supervisor cannot stop there. Supervisors must become accomplished in the art of effective employee relations, which is the practice of preventing a need for unionization. As many supervisors in unionized hospitals will attest, supervision with a union contract is significantly more difficult. It behooves the health care supervisor to practice good employee relations, thus precluding the need for employees to seek third-party representation.

This chapter will first address the preventive measures a supervisor must practice to avoid having to share some of his authority with the union through its shop stewards and negotiated contract. Later in the chapter, labor relations and the implications of the 1974 health care amendments to the NLRA will be discussed.

EMPLOYEE RELATIONS

Prior to discussing labor relations and the various facets of the National Labor Relations Act, particularly with regard to the various implications it has for the supervisor in a decentrally managed organization, it is perhaps appropriate to turn our attention to employee relations, which is the art and practice of treating employees with respect and dignity.

Good employee relations must be practiced each day. Much of the unionization in the health care field today is attributable to supervisors who have somehow failed to develop some expertise in human relations. Instead of developing an ongoing, honest, caring relationship with their employees and treating them as equals, these supervisors are practicing authoritarian styles of leadership. During a union organizational attempt, more often than not employees are voting not for or against the union but for or against the type of supervision they receive.

Being an efficient and effective supervisor requires many talents. Fortunately, most of these talents can be acquired by a combination of education, experience, and the desire to do a better job. In order to fully understand employee relations, let us first take a look at how the union organizing campaign gets started.

CAUSES OF UNION ORGANIZATION CAMPAIGNS

The collective bargaining process must be viewed as the means to an end and not the objective in and of itself. Employees use the unionization process as a means to gain what they have failed to gain any other way, be it respect from their supervisors, better wages, working conditions, or whatever. Unionization is not sought just for the sake of unionization. The management must learn to provide avenues for change within the institution so that employees won't have to seek outside (third-party) intervention. Unfortunately, the management in health care institutions has traditionally waited to react to outside forces. It is time to take the initiative within the organization and develop the means for the management and the workers to relate to each other with mutual good faith.

Supervisors must be sensitive to employee needs since union organizing action is usually initiated by an unsatisfied employee or group of employees. For example, employees who have repeatedly asked for repairs to the locker room facilities, improved scheduling to prevent long work stretches, or improved leadership and have received either no reply or an unsatisfactory reply are employees who will seek that outside means to have their needs and concerns heard and dealt with once and for all.

A lot of research has been undertaken on the major causes of job dissatisfaction. As every institution differs, so do the various needs and concerns of the employees. Many institutions attempt to evaluate employee discontent through employee attitude surveys. These surveys, often many pages in length, ask each employee many questions about the job, the supervisor, and the institution. Through an analysis of the results, major areas of concern can be discovered and hopefully alleviated by the management.

Certain factors consistently show up in these surveys and can be grouped into three major classifications. The first is poor supervision or leadership, as exhibited by a supervisor who is inflexible and authoritarian and who doesn't permit employee participation in departmental decision making or goals. The second is lack of communication. Supervisors must function as leaders, and they have only one basic instrument by which they can coordinate the various activities of their employees and transform them into an efficient working operation. That instrument is communication. The third is unsafe or poor working conditions, be it leaky faucets in the bathrooms, broken windows in the maintenance shop, or questionable understaffing in a patient care unit.

Specialists in employee relations believe that union organizing activity in a health care facility can be only rarely explained by a single identifiable cause of dissatisfaction. They believe instead that employees gravitate toward a union when their overall feelings about their jobs and working conditions are negative. Many elements, as we can see, enter into an employee's attitude about his or her job. And different employees, of course, may be motivated by different factors. Union campaigns get started when at least some of the following factors are answered *no* by several employees. Do the employees believe that

1. they are regularly treated with courtesy, respect, and dignity?
2. they are treated as individuals, with unique needs, skills, and aspirations?
3. the management makes personnel decisions fairly without regard to race, sex, age, religion, nationality, or the like?
4. their supervisors are careful to avoid favoritism in directing work, imposing discipline, and dispensing rewards?
5. their efforts and loyalty are known and appreciated?
6. the management voluntarily grants reasonable, competitive wage increases and improves employee benefits?
7. day-to-day working relationships are friendly and relaxed?
8. their workplaces are attractive, healthy, and safe?
9. their jobs are secure from unwarranted discharge?
10. their work is genuinely important to the welfare of patients and the community?
11. they have received adequate training to enable them to perform well?
12. the institution itself is managed in a highly professional manner?
13. their jobs hold promise for a better future, with opportunities to upgrade skills, enjoy greater responsibility, and achieve higher earnings?

If these questions can be answered affirmatively, employees will have little interest in union representation.

Unfortunately, due to the manner in which the NLRA is written, as we shall examine in greater depth later in this chapter, the union organizer can come along and *promise* to correct all the inadequacies and deficiencies that the employee perceives to be present. The management, on the other hand, can promise *nothing* during an organizational attempt lest it be construed as an "unfair labor practice." Union organizers are people-oriented; they communicate well with workers. They look at the workers' side of the issues and are sympathetic to their feelings. In short, they become everything a supervisor isn't. Employees thus become attracted to them and pledge their support to further the union cause. Union organizers are trained in the techniques of motivation; unfortunately, supervisors are not.

The organizer knows how to appeal to employees. Organizers are tuned to the desires hidden behind employees' many vocal complaints. The union organizer will promise to protect employees from unjust discharge and discipline and to install, through a union contract, a grievance procedure as well as a defined disciplinary process, if either is lacking. The organizer will appeal to the need of employees for economic gains and will promise better wages and employee benefits through a union contract. "Wages will be competitive not only locally but also regionally, particularly with larger union hospitals," promises the organizer.

Employees who are often intimidated by their supervisors will feel comfort in the fact that the union organizer also promises to act as the employees' agent against that "big bad person." The union will act in the employees' behalf and will act as insulation between the workers and the management. Also contained within the union message is the statement that there is strength in numbers. Collectively, employees can have a voice in decision making. Their union contract will allow them to stand together and give them the strength to be treated with the respect and dignity they deserve.

Those experienced in employee/labor relations matters confirm one basic method of effectively and successfully maintaining good employee relations. This method is called *reality*. Unless the supervisor has some way of finding out what reality is, there is no way he or she can maintain a good relationship with employees. A sound two-way communication system is the key to reality. Reality consists of employee sentiments, feelings, gripes, grievances, desires, ambitions, needs, and wants. Reality also includes the following.

Listening (do not confuse with interrogation)

Listening uncovers clues that explain absenteeism, turnover, reasons for poor performance, patient complaints, low productivity, health problems, and so on. It must be part of a regular system, and it requires a flexible, alert management that has learned how to make adjustments and corrections quickly where required. Listen to employees, but more importantly, hear what they are saying. Try to understand their problems and concerns by placing yourself in the employee's situation.

Promotions

If a new job opens up, current employees should be given every opportunity for that job—even if it requires extra training and costs. Post jobs and develop career ladders within your department and the institution. Above all, dare to give up that good employee to another department.

Transfers

The supervisor should permit second- and third-shift employees to transfer to a more convenient shift instead of hiring someone off the street to work the desired shift. Don't sabotage promotions or transfers from within the facility.

Discipline

Although this item is discussed at length in the next chapter, certain points are essential to our understanding of sound employee relations. All too often, when we think of discipline we think of punishment. Actually, discipline should not be equated with punishment; it should be educational for both the worker and the supervisor. It is far better to use this "clinical approach" to discipline rather than to view discipline as punishment. A supervisor should help an employee understand why his or her behavior is contrary to agreed-upon standards or existing policy. Get the facts. Why did the employee fail to perform? Why did the employee act as he or she did? Are there any contributing factors—personal, family, peer-relationship, etc.? Plan to talk with your employees—an informal, friendly talk.

Grievances

Grievances should represent problems to be solved, not agreements to be won. Make sure the problem is well defined and that you are solving the problem and not a symptom of the problem. Don't hold a grudge against any employee who files a grievance, even if that grievance is directed against you personally. When it comes to resolving a grievance, do not wait until you have spare time. Grievance procedures usually guard against this, since set time limits for resolving the problem are prescribed. However, when an employee comes to a supervisor with a specific problem or concern, it may quite frequently be brushed aside and dealt with when all other things are done. Decision making within the grievance procedure must be done in an orderly, uniform manner. Maintain the integrity of the grievance procedure at all times; at no time should you make short-term decisions to ease the problem at hand. Examine the consequences of your decision and how it will affect you and your department in the future. Decisions that are made should be uniform for all employees, and, as in other areas, don't show favoritism. Of the challenges facing supervisors today, consistency is perhaps one of the greatest. Maintaining consistency in your every action is difficult to achieve, but by striving for it you will ultimately improve your effectiveness as a supervisor. Past experience has shown that supervisors who are consistent are regarded by top management as better supervisors, and they do in fact have less employee relations problems. In short, it pays to be consistent; it makes your job that much easier. When it comes right down to it—when you're resolving a grievance—don't ever be afraid to admit your own mistakes.

Supervisor attitude

A preschool child put in front of the television screen learns the importance of the two expressions "please" and "thank you." For reasons not fully understood at this time, these simple expressions of human relations seem to be ignored by adults and specifically supervisors. The employee is told, not asked, to perform, and there is little sense of appreciation expressed. The employee senses exploitation rather than a recognition of the dignity of the individual. Having lived through the 1960s, now referred to as the "era of personhood," employees (particularly those of the younger generation) have been exposed to equal rights, civil rights, women's rights, and equal-employment-opportunity rights. The importance of the individual is emphasized in such union campaign slogans as "I am somebody." The employee wants to be identified as an individual entitled to dignity.

An employee stated recently in a morale survey, "I don't care how much you know until I know how much you care." The emphasis today should be on a sincere, concerned, and caring relationship between the management and its work force.

Communication is the basis of human relationships. Until there is effective communication, there is no relationship. Once the relationship is established, however, it is vital that it be maintained with consistency and sincerity.*

Supervisory conduct

Supervisors, in order to get things done with other people, must learn to get along with others. The following section offers helpful guidelines.

How to get along with others

1. Keep skid chains on your tongue. Say less than you think. Cultivate a pleasant voice. How you say it is often more important than what you say.
2. Make few promises and keep them faithfully, no matter what the cost.
3. Never let an opportunity pass to give a well-deserved compliment.
4. If criticism is needed, do it tactfully.
5. Be interested in others—their work, their homes and families. Let everyone you meet feel that you regard them as a person of importance.
6. Don't burden or depress those around you by dwelling on your minor aches and pains and small disappointments. Everyone has to deal with something in life that is not exactly as he or she would like it to be.
7. Discuss, don't argue.

---

*"Supervisor Attitude" is adapted from a section on pp. 50–51 in W. I. Christopher, "Positive Supervisory Practices to Maintain Nonunion Status in a Hospital," in Joseph J. Bean, Jr., and Rene Laliberty, *Understanding Hospital Labor Relations: An Orientation for Supervisors*, Reading, Massachusetts: Addison-Wesley, 1977, pp. 41–53.

8. Let your virtues, if you have any, speak for themselves. Don't indulge in gossip. It's a waste of time and can be destructive.
9. Be respectful of the feelings of others. Wit and humor at the expense of a friend is rarely worth the small laugh, and it may hurt more than you know.
10. Pay no attention to derogatory remarks about you. The person who carried the message may not be the world's most accurate reporter.
11. Do your best to forget about the rewards. If you deserve credit, someone will "remember." Success is much sweeter that way.
12. Keep in mind that the true measure of an individual is how well he or she treats a person who cannot return the favor.

Participation

Everyone wants to have some say in what affects them. Supervisors have to learn to involve employees in the operation of their departments. Ask yourself, "Why can't the employees help make the decision? Why can't the employees help evaluate the alternatives to problems?" If you have a specific problem, learn to involve employees in helping you to define and analyze it and in developing various alternative solutions. You have to learn to create a team relationship with your subordinates. In achieving greater participation of employees in departmental affairs, you will be making the employee part of the solution process and not part of the problem.

The management has a better opportunity to succeed in their endeavors by creating a team relationship with the employee, seeking his or her advice, and asking for recommendations. Working together to fulfill common objectives can create a true sense of community or team spirit. A team wins together or loses together; it is not composed of some winners and some losers. The extent to which real team recognition can be achieved is one important means of minimizing the eventual obstructionism and the separation of the managers and employees into opponents destined for confrontation.

There are other ways of developing good employee relations. The following points are suggested.

Recognize any insulation between you and your employees.

- When employees have nonwork problems do they (a) usually talk to you? (b) usually turn to co-workers? (c) or are you not sure what they do?
- How do employees learn your opinion of their performance? (a) They are told when they do wrong. (b) You have regular discussions with them. (c) You really don't know.

- How do you keep your people informed? (a) You tell them what they need to know. (b) You hold regular group or individual meetings. (c) You communicate primarily with memos.

(Best answers: first (a), second (b), third (b). Other answers mean that there is insulation.)

Get to know your staff.
Develop a "profile" of each employee.

- List the name of each person under your direction.
- Jot down each person's interests, background, and work needs (research and discussion may be necessary).
- Develop the art of listening.

Just as patient care plans are developed for our patients, so should employee care plans be developed for your employees.

Let your staff know you.

- Don't hold back from discussing or commenting on nonwork matters.
- Congeniality doesn't breed contempt. Employees like to know your interests.
- Maintain your visibility at all levels of management. Get around; visit departments and employees.

Let your staff in on things.

- Tell them individually or in groups what's going on throughout the hospital.
- Spend five minutes each day discussing work matters with an employee (a small investment that pays big dividends).
- Share with them your new plans and the ideas being discussed; listen to their views.

Build your credibility.

- Be decisive, and explain your reasons.
- Get the facts before reprimanding or criticizing (practice constructive criticism).
- Give an employee the benefit of doubt.
- Don't pass the buck when reporting a negative decision.
- Practice consistency when applying rules and policies.
- Know the personnel policies of the hospital.
- Know the wage/benefit program.
- Be willing to admit it when you've made a mistake.

- Know where to refer problems.
- Don't forget to follow up quickly on situations brought to your attention.
- Don't forget to feed back information relative to employees' suggestions.
- Conduct your annual performance evaluations promptly.

LABOR RELATIONS AND THE 1974 HEALTH CARE AMENDMENTS TO THE NATIONAL LABOR RELATIONS ACT

What happens if the positive employee relations methods discussed above are not put into practice? The dissatisfied employee may seek out the union to represent him or her, to get what the management has failed to provide. An understanding of the National Labor Relations Act and the implications it has for you is required.

First, it is vitally important to realize that under the NLRA, supervisors are not considered employees of their particular institutions; rather, they are part of the management. Although many supervisors are taken by surprise by this statement, the reasons are quite clear when one understands the purpose of the law.

Laws are generally written to protect the rights and privileges of both parties. The NLRA was designed to distinguish and regulate the relationship between employees and employers. Therefore, it becomes necessary to identify who is labor and who is management. Hence, for labor relations purposes under the NLRA, supervisors are managers, not employees, and are exempt from the act. To be exempt as a supervisor, the individual must have the authority to hire, transfer, suspend, lay off, recall, promote, discharge, assign, reward, or discipline other workers, or to have the "responsibility to direct," or to adjust grievances, or to effectively command such action. But the supervisor need not have all these powers; supervisors can be exempt if they have any one of them.

Because supervisors as defined above are considered part of the management, the restrictions placed upon the management by the act become "an inherited supervisory legacy." Supervisors must realize that they are part of the management, in their every action, in their spoken word.

Any understanding of the NLRA is not complete unless the supervisor understands what it actually says. The NLRA is broken down into various subsections of law. Section I contains a very important policy statement. It explains quite clearly that the purpose of the law is to encourage employees in their efforts to organize and to protect them in those efforts. Not stated but implied is assistance to unions in the organizing of employees and encouragement for collective bargaining. This is the premise of the entire law, and it is unfair to a great degree. There is a double standard running throughout this law. At numerous times during an organizational attempt, events will occur in which the union or the union organizer will be able to do certain things, but you, as part of the management, can't.

Section II contains some very important definitions. For instance, what is an employee? What is a supervisor? What is a labor organization?

Sections III through VI define the National Labor Relations Board. The board itself has two major functions. The first is to conduct secret ballot elections in appropriate bargaining units. The second is to adjudicate unfair labor practices.

Section VII is largely the essence of the act. Employees have the right to self-organize, to form, join, or assist labor organizations, and to engage in other concerted activities for the purpose of collective bargaining. As a result of this section, employees also have the right to refrain from any or all of this activity.

Some key words appear in Section VII of the NLRA. Concerted activities pertain not only to union activities but also to nonunion group activities. Concerted nonunion group activity can be said to happen when two or more employees act together as a group for mutual aid or protection. It is important to note that a concerted activity does not have to be a union activity to be protected under the NLRA. Concerted activity includes such things as a presentation of a grievance in a group or on behalf of a group of employees, a sick-out by two or more employees to protest pay, work schedules, or unsafe conditions, group meetings to request a wage increase, picketing to protest employers' racially discriminatory hiring practices, and employees protesting employers' noncompliance with any federal law on wages, hours, and working conditions. As concerted activities, they are protected under the NLRA. Therefore, supervisors must be reminded of unfair labor practices while dealing with these activities.

An interesting case in point regarding concerted activities recently occurred. Mercy Hospital Association, Inc., was cited for acting unlawfully when it fired *nonunionized* nurses who walked out to protest an administrator's refusal to hear their grievance. The NLRA gives employees the right to engage in concerted activities for collective bargaining or other mutual aid or protection. Despite what many of us believe, this applies to nonunionized as well as unionized employees. The case in question involved a hospital walkout. Objecting to the fact that the number of nurse's aides on their shift was reduced from eight to five, six nurses tried to voice their displeasure to the hospital administrator. When he sent them word that he would not see them, they walked out. The hospital, citing their unauthorized absences and their failure to first use the required ("unilateral") grievance procedure, fired them. The NLRB said that the discharge of nonunionized employees engaged in the spontaneous work stoppage infringed on their right to engage in protected concerted activities. The right to engage in a strike or concerted work stoppage could not be circumvented by a company rule prohibiting employees from leaving work without permission. Noting that the one day walkout did not cause an emergency at this hospital, the board ordered reinstatement and back pay (*Mercy Hospital Association, Inc.*, 235 N.L.R.B. 97 (1978)).

Special restrictions apply to union employees in health care institutions, because work stoppages might result in life-threatening situations. Unions must give the management advance notice of any intent to stop work. However, in this instance the board said that these restrictions did not apply because these concerted activities were by nonunionized hospital workers and there had been no emergency caused by the walkout. The board presumably might have had a different decision if patient care had been in jeopardy. Your right to discipline or fire workers for disruptive conduct can be considerably restricted if their action falls into the concerted activity category.

Closely aligned with these concerted activities are the "unfair labor practices" (ULPs), which are in Sections VIIIA and VIIIB of the NLRA. Section VIIIA lists the employer ULPs, while Section VIIIB lists the union ULPs. Section VIIIB, if one looks at a copy of this law, is twice as long as Section VIIIA. However, don't let the length fool you. The great majority of ULP cases heard by the board are employer ULPs. ULPs constitute what you can and cannot do during a union organization attempt. Supervisors, during a period of attempted organization or, as was just pointed out, during concerted activity for mutual aid and protection, must be mindful of ULPs. Employer ULPs are best remembered by recalling the acronym TIPS; the management cannot Threaten, Interrogate, Promise, or Spy on union activities. The management can, however, give facts, state opinions, and give examples. To explain TIPS further, the management cannot threaten employees with loss of employment if the employee expresses support for a union. The management cannot ask employees to reveal the extent of union activity or union organizing occurring within the institution. The management cannot, for instance, promise a significant wage increase during an organization attempt, and it cannot spy on union organization activity. What the management can do is give facts about the union. "If you join the union you will have to pay union dues every month." The information you give must be factual. Dues must be quoted accurately. You must be able to substantiate the information about the union. You can state your opinion about unions and what the union's past history has been. You can give examples. For instance, you can say to your employees, "Here is a sample union security clause; if the union is voted in, you may be forced to join even if you didn't vote for it."

Section VIIIC of the act contains the "free speech doctrine"; it states the right of all parties, including the management, the union, and the worker, to express their views in written, oral, printed, and graphic forms. Section VIIID lists the ground rules for collective bargaining, which is basically the mutual obligation of the employer and the employee representatives to meet at reasonable times and to confer in mutual good faith. Section IX of the act sets forth the procedure for the representation election.

Since the NLRA was amended in 1974 to include nonprofit institutions, two items have caused considerable concern and have been in a constant state of flux. The first is the rule surrounding solicitation and distribution within institutions. In this area, employees have certain rights, which must be recognized and respected. It is perhaps appropriate to first define certain terms related to the solicitation and distribution rights of employees. Solicitation is defined as the practice, act, or instance of approaching an employee and asking him or her to take a certain action, for example, to sign an authorization card, support a particular cause, or whatever. Distribution, on the other hand, is the wholesale handing out of leaflets, handbills, and so on. Incidentally, the union authorization card is considered a form of solicitation and not a form of distribution. Outsiders are those people or those individuals who are not employed by the institution. Of course, employees are those individuals who are employed by the institution. Work time includes the working time of both the employee doing the soliciting and distributing and the employee to whom it is directed. Nonwork areas (where a substantial amount of the confusion surrounding solicitation and distribution has occurred) include places such as employee lounges, rest rooms, parking lots, stairways, cafeterias, canteens, sidewalks, and gift shops. Work areas are those areas not defined as nonwork areas. Simply stated, the general rules for solicitation and distribution are the following.

> Outsiders may not solicit for any purpose or distribute any literature on an institution's property at any time. Employees may not solicit for any purpose during working time and in working areas, and employees may not distribute any literature for any purpose during working time or in working space.

The first significant case involving solicitation and distribution was that of St. John's Hospital, Tulsa, Oklahoma. The NLRB ruled in March 1976 that by prohibiting union solicitation and distribution by employees during their nonworking time in employee-only working areas as well as patient access areas such as cafeterias, lounges, hallways, coffee shops, and the like, the hospital had violated the NLRA (*St. John's Hospital and School of Nursing, Inc.*, 222 N.L.R.B. 182 (1976)). However, in July 1977 the U.S. Court of Appeals for the Tenth Circuit overturned a significant part of the board decision (*St. John's Hospital and School of Nursing, Inc. v. NLRB*, 82 Lab. Cas. Para. 10,021 (10 Cir. July 14, 1977)). Although the court sustained the board's order to permit employee solicitation in employee-only working areas, where there is no mingling of patients and employees, the court reversed the board's decision regarding patient access areas. Briefly, the court ruled that all areas of the hospital to which patients have access must be areas that the hospital is entitled to regulate. Thus hospitals have the right to prohibit solicitation in areas where there is a mingling of staff (employees) and patients. For example, if a hospital's cafeteria and gift shop were both open to the public, they certainly would be restricted with respect to solicitation and distribution.

The court's decision is highly significant for hospitals, since it provides judicial authority for hospitals that adopt a rule preventing solicitation and distribution in all areas of the institution to which patients, visitors, and the public have access. In contrast to the St. John's Hospital decision was the later case of *Beth Israel Hospital v. NLRB*, 98 S. Ct. 2463 (1978). This case was a final determination of whether the hospital had violated Section VIIIA1 of the NLRA by enforcing its no-solicitation rule. The rule banned employees from soliciting for the union and distributing union literature during nonworking time in all areas of the facility to which patients and visitors have access, including the cafeteria and coffee shop. This case arose because of the organization campaign of Local 88 of the Service Employees International Union at Beth Israel Hospital in Boston, during which an employee distributed union literature in the hospital cafeteria. When this employee was given a warning, the union filed a ULP charge. In this case, the Supreme Court of the United States unanimously rejected the claim of the hospital that the special needs of the hospital's patients justified a complete ban of employee solicitation and distribution of union literature in all areas of its facility accessible by patients and visitors, including the cafeteria and coffee shop. The Court noted that patients are not allowed to visit the cafeteria unless their doctors certify that they are well enough to do so. Thus patient use of the cafeteria is voluntary, random, and infrequent. It is of critical significance that only 1.56 percent of the cafeteria's patrons are patients. Accordingly, the Court maintained that the potential for disruption of patient care caused by solicitation and distribution in the cafeteria and coffee shop of this hospital was remote.

These two cases illustrate the fact that, depending on the circumstances that exist within your particular institution, enforcement of rules regarding solicitation and distribution can vary. When there is a mingling of patients, visitors, and staff, a hospital has every right to regulate solicitation and distribution. However, if the surrounding is similar to that in the Beth Israel case, there is only a slight possibility that there could be a mingling of staff with patients and visitors, and employees may have every right to solicit and distribute literature in that particular area.

The second major area of concern centers around "appropriate bargaining units." The National Labor Relations Board determines whether a particular group of employees constitutes an appropriate bargaining unit, that is, whether certain employees or groups of employees should be included together in a unit and be allowed to vote as a group for union representation. In keeping with the congressional mandate to prevent undue proliferation of bargaining units, the NLRB set forth in the summer of 1975 the following five broad categories of health care employees as appropriate bargaining units. The first was registered nurses, the second was other professionals, the third was all technical employees, the fourth was clerical employees, and the fifth was service and maintenance employees. However, because of various court and NLRB decisions since these original guidelines, modifications have been made in the delineation of potential bargaining units. The first major category now contains three bargaining units. The first unit contains registered nurses, the second contains all other residual professionals such as physical therapists and pharmacists, and the third contains the salaried medical doctors (not residents and interns, who are considered to be students of the institution). The second major category contains the technical staff, including licensed practical nurses, X-ray technicians, inhalation therapists, and so on.

The third major category contains business office clerical employees, excluding medical-record file clerks, transcriptionists, and medical secretaries, who fall into the fourth category, service and maintenance. Because of inconsistent NLRB decisions, the fourth category is a catch-all unit that is the largest of all hospital appropriate bargaining units. However, by law the security guards constitute a separate unit. Boiler operators have also been found to be a separate appropriate bargaining unit. In addition, there may have been units formed resulting from earlier bargaining history, as well as units of the state labor relations board set up prior to the 1974 amendments to the NLRA. There could also be units which are stipulated in an agreement between the employer and union. As a result of all this, the five originally intended categories of appropriate bargaining units has now mushroomed to between ten and fifteen appropriate bargaining units in a hospital, each with its own separate interest.

Now that we know what constitutes an appropriate bargaining unit, attention must be turned to the representation election and the process by which that election takes place. There is normally a considerable amount of organizing activity occurring within your institution prior to the election. This activity could be occurring either with or without the supervisor's knowledge. Once this organizational activity has reached a level acceptable to the union, the institution may well receive what is called a "recognition demand letter," in which the union states that it represents a majority of the employees in appropriate bargaining units. The union asks the top management of the institution to recognize the union as the sole bargaining agent for employees within an appropriate bargaining unit. What top management usually does, after conferring with its legal counsel, is to instruct the union to file an election petition or representation petition with the appropriate regional office of the NLRB and to request a secret ballot election. The institution usually denies that the union does, in fact, represent a majority of the employees in a particular unit. The union then files a representation petition with the appropriate regional office of the NLRB.

Once the petition is received by the NLRB, the regional director of the board advises the employer by letter that a petition has been filed and encloses with that letter a copy of the petition, a poster outlining employer and employee rights and obligations under the NLRA, and a questionnaire to determine the extent of the institution's coverage under the NLRA. The regional director also states that the union apparently has a sufficient "showing of interest" if that union possesses signed authorization cards from 30 percent of the employees in a potential bargaining unit. The director requests that the employer send an alphabetical listing of employees within the potential bargaining unit to determine whether this 30 percent showing of interest actually exists. A hearing is then scheduled. This normally takes place 30 days after the receipt by the employer of the petition copy sent from the NLRB.

The institution has two major strategy decisions during the hearing. The first is to question the appropriateness of the unit. The second is the timing of the election. Once these two factors are determined, an election agreement is reached, an election date is set, and the unit appropriateness is determined. The institution is then requested by the NLRB to supply the board with what is called an "excelsior list," which is a list of names and addresses of all employees in the appropriate bargaining unit. The purpose of this list, of course, is to allow the union greater access to the employees within that particular unit. It is generally given to the union at least two weeks prior to the election. Also contained within the board's request for the excelsior list is the election notice itself. The election notice must be posted throughout the institution. It explains where and when the election is going to be held and who is eligible to vote in the election.

The election itself is conducted by secret ballot, as done for political elections in democratic countries. At the election, there are numerous observers from both the union and the management sides, and a National Labor Relations Board agent is also present. Employees file into the election place, have their names checked against the master voting list, mark their ballot secretly, and deposit it in a ballot box. The election results are determined by a simple majority of those voting. For example, if an appropriate bargaining unit contains 60 employees who all vote and if 31 employees vote for the union, the union will triumph.

Suppose only 30 of 60 employees voted; if 16 voted for the union, the union would again win and would then be the duly elected representative of the entire 60 people in the appropriate bargaining unit. It is readily apparent that supervisors must encourage *all* employees to vote in the election.

To conclude, it is important to note that employees usually vote for or against their immediate supervisor rather than for or against top management, the Board of Trustees, or whomever. Through its actions the management can drive employees into unions. The management may allow certain inequities to exist, and the union takes the opportunity to provide a means for the worker to retaliate against the management.

Employees who sense appreciation for their efforts will not seek a union. The employee who has a sense of confidence in his or her management and works in an environment of productive and satisfying human relationships will not turn to an outside "third party" for representation. The responsibility for preventing outside representation rests with the supervisor; the choice rests with the worker.*

Did you know that *unions represent 20 percent of hospital workers?* Voluntary union members amount to 16.6 percent, according to 1977 figures released in June 1979 by the Department of Labor's Bureau of Labor Statistics. The balance, 3.4 percent, are involuntary members by virtue of security-clause arrangements. The 20 percent figure represents 719,000 workers in the hospital industry as of May 1977. A total of 582,000 employees were found to voluntarily belong to unions. The balance of 137,000 pay dues involuntarily.

In public hospitals, 391,000 employees—35.7 percent—were represented by labor organizations, but only 13.7 percent were represented in private hospitals.

Average weekly earnings for hospital employees were $212 per week for those represented by unions and approximately $205 for those not represented. Men in the health industry made an average of $231 per week, while women averaged $202.

*Paragraph adapted from Christopher, p. 53.

the art of positive discipline

To each of us involved in the supervision of employees, discipline has different meanings and connotations. Discipline in its broadest sense means internal (departmental or work-unit) orderliness—the opposite of confusion. Discipline, as we shall use the term, does not mean strict and technical observance of rigid work rules and regulations. Discipline should mean workers cooperating, behaving and performing in a normal and orderly way on their own. The best discipline is self-discipline.

In the "good old days" discipline often failed to meet standards that were constructive or even fair. In fact, contrary to modern management theories, discipline has traditionally been both severe and irresponsible.

STANDARDS OF DISCIPLINE

Every supervisor must make sure that all disciplinary action taken

1. is fair;
2. is consistent with sound principles of personnel relations (including the right to appeal);
3. is in accordance with general institutional statements about discipline that are clear and familiar to everyone concerned; and
4. implements ideas that have been developed in consultation with those subject to disciplinary action.

Only when discipline meets these standards can it reasonably be expected to play a part in the kind of mutually responsible action that contributes to peak efficiency. It represents management by shared objectives.

In this chapter we will consider the following questions, which should be thought about by every supervisor. Why plan for disciplinary action? What needs to be said in an organizational discipline policy? What makes an organizational disciplinary procedure acceptable and workable? What steps should be included in the disciplinary process?

WHY PLAN FOR DISCIPLINARY ACTION?

Modern management theorists now believe that peak performance in every organization depends on action by which subordinates willingly carry out instructions and orders issued by supervisors and abide by rules of conduct and standards of work established to ensure the successful attainment of organizational objectives. According to this concept, effective discipline is a by-product of positive and intelligent leadership and of willing cooperation by subordinates. It exists within the framework that is provided by policies and procedures established and accepted for the organization as a whole. The discipline achieved is called constructive self-discipline.

If all employees could be counted on at all times to behave reasonably, there would be no need for supervisors to take disciplinary action. By the same token, if all supervisors could be counted on to be reasonable in imposing discipline, there would be no need to set up a procedure for disciplinary processes. Human nature being what it is, neither of these expectations is realistic.

Unfortunately, in a health care institution as in any organization there are likely to be a few employees who, for various reasons, fail to observe established rules and standards, even after having been informed of them.

THE NEGATIVE VIEW OF DISCIPLINE

Some supervisors still think of discipline only as punishment rather than as a form of education. Even today, they see it as a means to counteract antisocial tendencies in employees by applying external pressure rather than as a way to reinforce self-discipline and group discipline. They hope that punishment will be effective as a deterrent. Or, in some cases, they mete out penalties as a form of retributive justice. Discipline can and should be educational, both on the part of the employee and on the part of the supervisor.

WHAT NEEDS TO BE SAID IN AN ORGANIZATIONAL POLICY FOR DISCIPLINE?

We strongly support the view that the primary purpose of discipline is to supplement and strengthen positive forces in the individual and his or her group. The following sample policy statement is an example of this approach.

> It is the intention of the management to promote at all times and throughout the whole employment relationship the high morale that leads to self-discipline in every employee and group discipline within every work team. When it is necessary for supervisors to resort to discipline, such action should demonstrably implement two related purposes: (1) to inform, remind, and encourage employees with regard to accepted standards of work and of conduct, and (2) to prevent an unruly minority from exercising an undue influence on standards of behavior.

In other words, whenever possible, the disciplinary procedure should be used in such a way and at such a time as to reinforce in employees the desire and ability to meet accepted standards of work and of conduct. Punitive action such as discharge should be taken only as a last resort. If there is doubt about the facts, suspension should be used pending further investigation.

Before we consider questions of disciplinary procedure, two comments on disciplinary policy seem in order. The first concerns having a minimum of rules. It is good policy to have as few rules as possible. A multiplicity of rules often breeds contempt for the very idea of law. Such contempt is usually expressed in nonobservance and nonenforcement of whatever rules are regarded as unimportant.

A second point to be noted about the sample disciplinary policy quoted above is that it does not include any comprehensive statement of disciplinary procedure. The disciplinary procedure is developed and issued separately. The policy thus becomes more durable; it will not change as specific rules for action are revised, and it provides broad guidelines for decision making.

WHAT MAKES AN ORGANIZATIONAL DISCIPLINARY PROCEDURE ACCEPTABLE AND WORKABLE?

No matter what else may be aimed at in a written statement of disciplinary procedure, two objectives are commonly agreed on. Firstly, the official statement should inform everyone concerned what top management expects (positively or negatively) of all employees. Employees cannot reasonably be expected to meet standards or to obey rules unless they know what the standards and rules are. Nor can supervisors be expected to represent top management in explaining and enforcing regulations without specific guidance. Thus there is a need to communicate what the rules are and what is expected of the employees.

Secondly, without uniformity of application, the same offense is almost certain to get different treatment at different times in different parts of the institution. Naturally, to formulate such a procedure is a responsibility of higher management, but its effectiveness depends on understanding and agreement at every organizational level, particularly the supervisory level. Uniform application of institutional rules and regulations is difficult to achieve; however, this must be our constant goal.

WHAT SHOULD BE SAID IN THE WRITTEN PROCEDURE?

Naturally, no list of offenses or rules can be comprehensive. A hospital-wide procedure resembles a hospital policy to the extent that its reference is necessarily general (although a procedure should be less general than a policy). Rules should be stated positively. Frequently, personnel handbooks are written in a style such as "Employee shall not . . ." or "Employees are not allowed to . . . ."

In hospitals where top management has a positive policy for discipline, the written procedure can suitably be stated as a general description of what employees are expected to do. An example of an appropriate written procedure follows.

> Everyone is expected to abide by all safety regulations and to be safety-conscious at all times, not only for himself or herself but also in relation to fellow employees. Every subordinate is expected to support management authority by following the instructions and obeying the orders issued by his or her immediate supervisor. Every employee should always show a responsible attitude toward work and toward other employees by reporting for work promptly and regularly and not leaving early, by meeting established standards for quantity and quality of work, by refraining from drinking intoxicating liquor or using controlled drugs, and by not offering such liquor or drugs to another employee.

Employees should be informed about rules

Whatever rules are adopted by the hospital, it is essential that employees be clearly informed about them. An effective kind of written communication is the employee handbook, in which a section can be devoted to summarizing or listing rules of conduct, the reasons for them, and, if desirable, the penalties that will result from violations.

THE DISCIPLINARY PROCESS

An effective disciplinary procedure should contain some statement about the kind of disciplinary action that will be taken when necessary. It is approved procedure in discipline cases that this action be made clear to all new employees before they become subject to discipline.

The question "What is disciplinary action?" is one that is answered differently in different hospitals and other businesses even today. But in an increasing number of cases, supervisors, personnel directors, and labor relations directors accept the concept that the disciplinary process not be restricted to official reprimands and other penalties. Instead, it should implement the analytical and educational approach and include all the following steps.

1. Preliminary investigation
2. An informal, friendly talk
3. An oral warning or reprimand
4. A written or official warning
5. A series of penalties such as disciplinary layoff, demotional downgrading or transfer, and, as a last resort, discharge

In addition to these steps, which *always* need to be taken (except when immediate discharge is warranted), another procedure that is sometimes desirable is suspension pending investigation. A sample suspension policy would read as follows.

> In disciplinary cases involving violation of hospital or departmental policies and procedures in which all of the facts cannot be promptly established, any member of the administration or a department head or supervisor can temporarily suspend an employee pending investigation. A suspended employee shall not be permitted to return to work until the matter is investigated and resolved by the department head and the Personnel Director. Such investigation shall include an interview with the suspended employee that should be completed promptly (no later than 5 days after the suspension date). Suspended employees shall not be paid during the suspension period and shall not be eligible for paid vacation time, sick time, or holiday time.

PRELIMINARY INVESTIGATION: GETTING THE FACTS

When a subordinate fails to meet established standards of work or of conduct, the first-line supervisor cannot afford to ignore or overlook this unsatisfactory behavior. The supervisor who accepts substandard work performance or condones breaches of conduct is communicating to employees that the announced rules and regulations are merely words. In fact, laxity of rule enforcement is often cited by offenders as an excuse. Unfortunately, this laxity is present all too often. If an employee has violated a work rule, make sure you don't ignore or overlook this behavior.

On the other hand, a supervisor should also refrain from taking hasty and perhaps unwarranted corrective action. Instead, when a breach of discipline occurs, just as when a piece of equipment breaks down, an alert supervisor investigates the reasons. Why did the employee fail to perform or act as he or she did? What hospital policies are involved, and more importantly, were they clearly understood by the employee? Has the employee's past record been spotty or is this the first offense? Are there any contributing factors such as ill health, family troubles, or an unsettled grievance that may explain this conduct? Here the capable supervisor is "getting down to cases." In most instances where discipline initially seems necessary, a brief preliminary investigation by the supervisor is the only action needed.

THE INFORMAL, FRIENDLY TALK

The informal, friendly talk is closely related to other supervisory techniques such as counseling and performance appraisals by which a supervisor helps subordinates to evaluate their current behavior with regard to agreed-upon standards. When the interview is part of the disciplinary process, aims should include getting at the reasons behind undesirable behavior, stimulating the sense of responsibility (which has not been evidenced by the employee), and perhaps strengthening or reestablishing the cooperative relationship that has been temporarily weakened or broken.

Such results are not always possible to achieve, but whatever the immediate outcome of the interview, the supervisor should never lose his or her temper or place the employee on the defensive.

If a friendly talk is not enough to create the desired result in employee behavior, the next step must be taken.

AN ORAL WARNING OR REPRIMAND

At this stage the possibility of imposing a penalty is specifically mentioned to the employee, but even so, disciplinary action remains unofficial to the extent that it need not become a matter of written record. The preventive purpose of discipline should still be stressed by the manner, tone, and wording of what has to be said. If a supervisor believes that no penalty needs to be imposed, that attitude can usually be communicated. On the other hand, if he or she looks forward to "getting" a subordinate whose behavior has been annoying, that feeling is almost certain to be detected—and resented—by the employee.

A tactful, friendly supervisor looks for a favorable time and place for such a talk, which should always be private. The aim is to help the employee correct his or her behavior by giving notice that poor work or undesirable conduct cannot be tolerated. The employee must be told that unless improvement is shown, he or she will be subject to official disciplinary action.

A WRITTEN WARNING OR REPRIMAND

If an employee does not respond to preliminary and unofficial talks in private, official disciplinary action is then called for. An official document should be issued. Hospitals should have a written warning notice; see Exhibit 9-1. The warning notice contains a statement of the offense and is to be signed by the employee. What if the employee refuses to sign? Refusal to sign represents a protest against the disciplinary action and may set the grievance process in motion, if the employee wishes to

EXHIBIT 9-1

WRITTEN WARNING

Date: _____

Name _____   Position _____

Supervisor's name _____

_____

SUPERVISOR'S DESCRIPTION OF INCIDENT:

_____

EMPLOYEE'S STATEMENT:

_____

DISCIPLINARY ACTION TAKEN:

_____

I acknowledge that the above
reprimand has been given to me.

_____   _____
Employee   Date   Supervisor   Date

                            _____
                            Department head   Date

cc: (Employee)   _____
    Personnel   Personnel Director   Date

file a grievance. In the event the employee does not wish to file a grievance, the person issuing the warning should date and initial it and include a written note stating that it has been reviewed with the employee, who refused to sign or file a grievance. A copy is sent to the Personnel Department, and a copy is given to the employee.

PENALTIES: UP TO AND INCLUDING DISCHARGE

In cases of repeated or continuing offenses or continuing failure to meet work standards, the supervisor is responsible for deciding what penalty is appropriate. A suitable penalty should be selected according to the seriousness of the offense and whether the undesirable action is a first, second, or third offense or a continuation of behavior about which the employee has been warned.

Termination of employment—the ultimate penalty

Discharge is such a drastic form of action that it should be reserved only for the most serious offenses or for people unresponsive to lesser penalties.

From the employee's standpoint, discharge represents a serious setback. It wipes out any seniority standing and makes new employment difficult to secure if the prospective employer learns why he or she left the last job. Moreover, since it reduces the chances of earning a livelihood, it may affect his or her personal and family relationships.

For a hospital or any other business, a discharge may involve serious losses and waste. Some of these losses can't be calculated strictly in terms of dollars. They include the time and money spent in hiring, training, and supervising an employee who now leaves the hospital. What can ultimately be more costly is the disruption of the work teams and the damage to morale occasioned by any discharge, especially if it is challenged. Further costs in money and morale result if a discharge results in a grievance that is processed all the way up to and through arbitration.

JUST CAUSE AND DUE PROCESS

The burden of proof for establishing "just cause" for discipline rests with the supervisor. Good cause must be shown for imposing disciplinary action, which means that supervisors may discipline only for sufficient and appropriate reasons. A second necessary ingredient in positive discipline is due process. An individual's right to due process is guaranteed in the Constitution of the United States. It involves four major steps.

DUE PROCESS

1. *Proper grounds for discipline* The supervisor has good cause and sufficient reason to discipline.
2. *Appropriate penalties* The discipline or supervisory action is appropriate to the severity of the work-rule violation.
3. *Fair play* In essence, consistency and uniformity regulate the application of work rules and discipline.
4. *Corrective procedure* The employee has been forewarned that his or her action is in violation of a work rule. The employee has been given a full *statement of charges* and also a *hearing*, which is an opportunity to present his or her side of the issue. Finally, the supervisor has observed any applicable time limits stated or implied in the disciplinary policy or procedure.

Coupled with the just cause and due process provisions is the right to appeal. Employees are to be afforded the opportunity to appeal any disciplinary action to a higher authority.

SUMMARY

Ideas about the exercise of management authority in disciplinary action have changed considerably since the "good old days." Arbitrary exercise of power is no longer tolerated in unionized work places, where management decisions have often been reversed by arbitrators because "due process" and "just cause" could not be proved. Discipline should be used primarily to reinforce self-discipline by individuals and work groups; penalties should be applied only after educational methods have failed.

A supervisor who believes that high morale and voluntary participation are prerequisites for peak efficiency naturally wishes to have a positive policy for discipline. Such a written policy can underline the desire of top management to ensure freedom from harassment for the cooperative majority and to guarantee the right of appeal for all.

The sequence of disciplinary steps that are specified as procedures followed by supervisors can exemplify the management's intent to use discipline primarily as a means of reeducation. For example, disciplinary action should start with a preliminary investigation in which a supervisor gets or checks facts to establish that someone is failing to meet reasonable requirements for work or conduct. In a case where the facts cannot be promptly established but the situation is potentially explosive, suspension is an appropriate alternative to discipline. The next two steps that are usually taken can both be informal. In a friendly talk, the supervisor can remind an employee about the purpose of a rule or the need for meeting standards. By following up with an unofficial warning if undesirable behavior is not corrected, the supervisor can underline the seriousness of a continuing disregard for organizational requirements. If these informal measures prove inadequate, official disciplinary action is not only justifiable but obligatory.

According to "due process," the first formal disciplinary step is to issue an official, written warning. If this warning is not heeded, a series of penalties begins. This series customarily starts with disciplinary demotion and proceeds to suspension and reclassification, finally reaching discharge—as a last resort!

achieving the objectives of the hospital by increased cooperation

This chapter will deal with the attainment of organizational objectives by planning on the departmental level. It also deals with managing change and the effect of change on teamwork, morale, supervisory behavior, and the work climate.

DEPARTMENTAL PLANNING

The time to plan today's job was yesterday.

Among the many so-called basic principles of management are unity of command, span of control, homogeneous assignment, and delegation of authority. Managers use the following basic methods in applying these principles: planning, organizing, directing, controlling, and coordinating.

So far as a supervisor is concerned, planning must be looked on as perhaps the most important of the five methods just named. It is very important that supervisors stay up to date with regard to changes affecting those supervised; planning must be in accordance with the supervisor's interpretation of the anticipated changes. It is just as important that the supervisor not wait too long before anticipated changes become effective. A well-administered department will not falter if properly alerted and prepared for changes. Any new assignment or change must not be made without due consideration for the people it will affect.

Planning is the primary task of every manager. Planning, as we use the term, is deciding in advance what is to be done in the future. Usually, it comes before any of the other managerial functions such as organizing, directing, controlling, and coordinating are carried out. In the planning process, the management is concerned about (1) the establishment of objectives to be attained and (2) determining how to achieve those objectives.

Planning is a continuous mental process. Therefore, it is necessary to think before you act and to act only in the light of facts, not guesses. Planning is the task of every manager and of every supervisor. However, prudent supervisors realize that they must avail themselves of all possible help when they undertake the planning process. For instance, in areas dealing with employee relations it is particularly helpful to discuss your plans and involve the Personnel Director in the planning process. Planning can also be a cost-savings measure because it prevents haphazard approaches and promotes an efficient and orderly operation.

What are some of the necessary steps in planning the work of a department?

1. Deciding what work is to be done
2. Determining the mission of the department
3. Understanding the purpose to be achieved by one and all
4. Deciding who is to do what elements of the work

5. Selecting new equipment that may be needed
6. Determining space requirements and planning layout with the building manager
7. Estimating the time needed
8. Estimating the staff necessary to achieve department objectives
9. Briefing everyone on their roles in the work to be done

How can supervisors plan for maximum results?

- Determine what *must be done*, what *ought to be done*, and what *need not be done.*
- Determine what elements of the work may safely be delegated to someone else.
- Schedule work to avoid a waste of both materials and the time and talents of the staff.
- Provide time for *advance planning.*
- Provide for flexibility.

In setting minimum and maximum goals for a department, the supervisor should be mindful of what goals can be expected and accepted. There is a need to decide what must be done now and what can be done later. Proper and appropriate planning consists of preparing not only for the job at hand but also for possibilities and probabilities.

ESTABLISHING DEPARTMENTAL GOALS

It is often said that effective management is always management by objectives. From our early training in the study of management, we may recall that there are two types of objectives, primary and secondary. Primary objectives are the overall objectives to be achieved by the institution. Usually, without primary objectives, no intelligent planning can take place. Primary objectives are the responsibility of top management such as the administration officers or the Board of Trustees.

Secondary objectives are the departmental goals. Since each department or section has a specific task to be performed, it follows that each must have its own clearly defined objective as a guide. Secondary objectives are always within the framework of the primary objectives and always contribute to the achievement of the primary objectives. Of course, secondary objectives are narrower in scope. The objectives of departments are somewhat more specific than primary objectives because they relate directly to departmental tasks.

Once departmental objectives are established, supervisors can develop plans which are necessary to achieve the objectives, i.e., which policies, procedures, methods, rules, regulations, and budgets to use. Each of these factors must be designed to reinforce one another.

PLANNING ON THE SUPERVISORY LEVEL

Planning, as we have stated, is deciding in advance what is to be done in the future. While the future remains uncertain, a supervisor must make certain assumptions about the future in order to plan. These assumptions are based on a forecast of what the future will hold. On a departmental level, a supervisor normally forecasts in two specific areas—technological developments and employee development and skills. Technological developments that may take place in the future could have a direct bearing on the way you carry out your departmental tasks. The area of employee development and skills concerns itself with the kinds of employees you will have working for you and perhaps an assessment of the need for upgrading certain employee skills and expertise.

It is the supervisor's duty to plan exactly how to utilize the available resources so that the work of the department can be carried out most effectively. A supervisor needs detailed plans on the utilization of equipment and tools, space, materials and supplies, and the time of both the supervisor and the employees.

Regarding tools and equipment, the supervisor needs to develop schedules both for replacement of worn-out or obsolete items and for preventive maintenance. Existing departmental space must be effectively utilized. The supervisor has to be constantly aware of the need to plan for improved departmental work flow and improved departmental layout. After labor, materials and supplies represent the most costly item. Supervisors must plan for the proper and effective use of materials and supplies, not only to prevent waste but also to improve departmental performance.

Time management should be a vital concern of every supervisor. Your time is a precious commodity. Keep the following tips in mind.

1. Don't procrastinate—learn to make up your mind without undue delay. However, don't make snap judgments.
2. Be specific—if someone wants to see you, don't say, "Anytime this week" or "Anytime this morning." Look at your calendar and schedule a specific time.
3. Watch the open door—don't kill the day by allowing employees to come in and "shoot the bull."
4. Don't trust your memory—always develop an "action list." Jot down reminders of things you need to do. Always carry a pocket notepad to jot down your reminders.
5. Use the exception principle—set a standard of production or work units or quality and let things be. Intervene only when an exception is obvious, such as when production drops below a certain level.

6. Delegate—examine what you do. Is it necessary for you to do this? Can it be eliminated? Can one of your employees do this task?

7. Think before you act—don't rush into action without first thinking and planning. Avoid doing something is haste merely to get a problem resolved.

8. Stay off the phone—try to limit your phone calls to three or four minutes. Talk business first, then chat about the baseball game or whatever.

9. Tackle the tough jobs first—don't postpone them. Do it at your peak of energy, which for many people is early in the morning.

10. Get the job started—even if you can't finish it, start it today and try to do a little each day.

11. Plan tomorrow today—projecting is the essence of planning. Look over what you have to do tomorrow. Then make plans about how it will be done, when it will be done, and who will do it.

12. Analyze your work every month—look at what you did. Can it be improved, eliminated, combined with other work, delegated?

13. Set aside some time to think each day—set some time aside without interruptions to plan your work, to improve your operations. Trying to work smarter, not harder, is the key. At the end of each day, review what you have done.

Achieving the objectives of the hospital requires the utilization of many skills, but first and foremost, the supervisor must learn to plan. Again, the time to plan today's job was yesterday.

MANAGING CHANGE

Progress requires change—changes in actions, ideas, attitudes, and knowledge. It's time for a change today, tomorrow, and the next day. Every day is a change day, whether we like it or not. It's no longer a question of whether there will be a change, but of how to ensure that changes will be implemented smoothly.

Every manager plays one of three roles during any change. He or she must act as a skillful implementer, suggester, or initiator.

The role of implementer is the most easy to understand. Your superior decides on a change and expects you, the manager, to carry it out. Sometimes you are convinced that it's a good change and enthusiastically implement it. If everyone concerned is enthusiastic, no problem occurs.

A dilemma arises, however, when you feel that the change dictated from above is not a good one. You must then decide whether or not to "enthusiastically" implement the change. In this case, you should question and challenge the suggested change. The additional information generated by further discussion may convince you of the change's value. If you remain unconvinced, the next approach is to discuss with your superior why you don't agree with the new plan. Your superior may show you that your skepticism is not justified. Or your superior may rescind or modify the change. If your superior insists that the change be made, you have only two choices—obey, or resist and suffer the consequences.

In the other two roles, you, as a manager, suggest or initiate the change. In both cases, the idea comes from yourself, a subordinate, or a peer not from your superior. Now you must decide whether to suggest the change to your boss or act on your own.

Several things determine which choice to make. The first is cost. If it is minimal, you can implement the change independently. If the cost is high, you should probably check with your superior. Another important consideration is how the change could affect other departments. Changes having possible widespread repercussions should be discussed with all parties concerned.

The third factor, probably the most significant one, has to do with the leadership style of your boss. Some superiors don't like to delegate authority. If this describes your boss, you should always suggest changes instead of initiating them. However, if your superior believes in the delegation of decision making, you are more free to initiate change.

Once the change is initiated, you must be prepared for at least some resistance to the new idea. People do not accept change for many reasons. Change disturbs the equilibrium of the current state of affairs. Employees are always comfortable with the present situation. They have worked themselves into a routine and are usually comfortable with it. They know what is expected of them, they know the work they have to do, and they feel confident of the way they are performing the work. Change is often viewed as a threat to the employee's security in several ways. The following is a list of reasons why employees resist change.

1. Insecurity—fear of failure and possibly losing job (may be realistic or unrealistic)
2. Habit—unwilling to break old habits
3. Antagonism toward person suggesting the change
4. Laziness—unwillingness to put forth effort to learn the new way
5. Loss of status—fear of becoming less important in eyes of other employees
6. Negative attitude toward job and/or organization
7. Does not feel involved—was not asked for an opinion about the change
8. Sees no need for change
9. Sees no good in change
10. Emotional reaction—doesn't like tone used by implementer

11. Implication of personal criticism—the new way implies the old way was not good (particularly if the old way was initiated by the person now on that job)
12. Economic uncertainty—change perceived as personal economic liability

On the other hand, employees accept and even welcome change for many reasons. Some of these reasons follow.

1. Personal benefit—will get better job, more money, more status
2. Positive attitude toward job and/or organization
3. Boredom—tired of present job, wants new challenge
4. Eagerness—shows initiative, cooperation, wants to get ahead
5. Respect for person implementing change
6. Necessity—feels change is needed
7. Involvement—suggested the change or had an opportunity to improve

HOW TO FACILITATE CHANGE

As the above list illustrates, employees seldom resist change just to be stubborn. Usually employees have what they consider valid arguments. The reasons for resisting or accepting change require you, the supervisor, to carefully manage and analyze each situation. The first requirement for successful implementation is to predict the resistance or acceptance on the part of those affected by your decision or by the change. This is called empathy, or "putting yourself in someone else's shoes." The second requirement is communications. Most resistance can be overcome by clearly and honestly communicating the reasons why—the reasons behind the change. This communicating should be done as far in advance as possible. By asking for ideas prior to the implementation of any change, you can get valuable information about how well the change will be accepted, as well as promoting greater acceptance. You have thus allowed employees to participate in the planning for change.

Participation can also be in the form of consultation, whereby criticism and suggestions are solicited from employees. In some instances, you can even let the employees make the decision regarding change themselves. Sometimes resistance can be overcome by moving very slowly.

Change is consistent, since it happens every day in some way. However, people's attitudes toward change are not consistent, whether those of superiors or subordinates. Working with these attitudes while making way for change is the challenge that every successful supervisor must confront and overcome.

TEAMWORK

Hospital objectives can be achieved only by mutual cooperation. Cooperation also depends on teamwork, which requires that people perform tasks together in working situations rather than just talk together. Following the old adage "the fellow in the boat with you never bores a hole in it," teamwork tries to get people in the boat rowing together.

There are some essential features of an operating team. A team requires a small, homogeneous group and a leader, someone who has accepted the responsibility of directing the group. A common objective is also required.

Teamwork requires regular interaction among the members of the team, and we must remember that we communicate only to the extent that we trust one another. Teamwork requires each member to contribute responsibly to the departmental objectives. A team spirit must be prevalent in the group, which requires a cooperative attitude. Everyone must be conscious of coordination. A group acts together as a team only after each person knows the social and functional roles of all others with whom he or she will be interacting.

As a supervisor, you can build a team relationship by developing a supportive environment. Like the mighty oak, teamwork grows very slowly, but on occasion it declines quickly, like that oak crashing to the forest floor. Therefore, supervisors should be mindful of how they design jobs and the responsibilities that they impose with jobs. Supervisors should also remember that in order to carry out work effectively and with high productivity, necessary capital equipment must be available.

The following list includes mistakes supervisors often make that cancel out cooperation.

Failing to keep people informed

Let people know where they stand. Let your close assistants in on your plans at an early stage. Let people know as early as possible of any changes that will affect them. Explain changes that will not affect them about which they may worry.

Failing to ask subordinates for their advice and help

Make them feel that your problem is their problem too. Encourage individual thinking. Make it easy for them to communicate their ideas to you. Follow through on their ideas.

Trying to be liked rather than respected

Don't do special favors trying to be liked. Don't try for popular decisions. Don't be soft about discipline, but maintain a sense of humor.

Failing to develop a sense of responsibility in subordinates

Allow freedom of expression. Give each person a chance to learn. When you give responsibility, also give authority. Hold subordinates accountable for results.

Emphasizing rules rather than skill

Give a person a job to do and then let him or her do it. Let an employee improve his or her own job methods.

Failing to keep criticism constructive

When something goes wrong, do you tend to assume who's at fault, or do you do your best to get all the facts first? Do you control your temper? Do you praise before you criticize? Do you listen to the other side of the story? Do you allow a person to retain dignity? Do you suggest specific steps to prevent recurrence of the mistake? Do you forgive and forget?

Not paying attention to employee gripes and complaints

(1) Make it easy for them to come to you. (2) Get rid of red tape. (3) Explain the grievance machinery. (4) Help a person voice his or her own complaint. (5) Always grant a hearing. (6) Practice patience. (7) Ask a complainer what he or she wants you to do. (8) Don't render a hasty or biased judgment. (9) Get all the facts. (10) Let the complainer know what your decision is. (11) Double-check your results. (12) Be concerned.

MORALE

Another item which greatly affects both the attainment of departmental objectives and cooperation is morale. The level of morale pertains to the spirit of a group and is to a great degree related to teamwork. Morale is the state of both mind and emotions involving the attitudes, feelings, and sentiments of individuals toward their work, environment, management, and peers.

Morale is not a single feeling; rather, it is a composite of feelings, sentiments, and attitudes. When morale is high, employees strive hard to accomplish the objectives of the department. When morale is low, it usually deters employees from the accomplishment of departmental objectives.

Morale is not something that is present or absent among employees. It is always present and by itself has neither favorable nor unfavorable meaning. Morale can range from excellent to poor. High morale is the result of good human-relations practices, which involve strong motivation and the management's respect for the dignity of the individual person.

In your day-to-day contact with employees as a supervisor, you can greatly influence and determine the level of morale. You must remember that maintaining the desired level of morale is a long-range project. It cannot be achieved solely on the basis of short-term devices such as pep talks, contests, or a slap on the back. However, morale is "contagious" and it can change very quickly.

Two major categories affect morale, external and internal factors. External factors are economic or personal problems and associations, such as car problems or sickness in the family. These items are normally beyond the scope of the supervisor and can only be dealt with indirectly. On the other hand, internal factors are items or conditions within the organization. Such things as appropriate incentives, good working conditions, and quality of supervision can all be directly affected by your actions as a supervisor. Good morale develops out of good human relations, which includes good employee motivation, respect for the individual, recognition of individual differences, good communication, understanding, and thoughtful counseling. As a supervisor, you have a responsibility to create a climate in which high morale will develop. Supervisors must learn to treat employees with the respect and dignity they deserve, recognizing that the employee is a person in his or her own right with individual differences, feelings, and desires. It is up to the supervisor to understand those feelings and desires and to channel them into productive pursuits, namely, achieving the organizational and departmental objectives.

techniques of interviewing and the selection process

The personnel work of a hospital should not be completely housed within the walls of one department. Personnel management is the responsibility of all department heads and people in supervisory positions.

What does the personnel function encompass? Despite many misconceptions, it does not include hiring and firing, which is the privilege and responsibility of the supervisor. The Personnel Director's role is to assist, by directing and guiding various activities through the supervisor to achieve a practical personnel program. In the employee-selection phase of personnel work, the Personnel Director hires no one, but does recruit, screen, and recommend applicants to the department head, who makes the final decision.

To assist you as a supervisor in the final decision of whether to accept or reject a recommended job applicant, you need a "tool"; thus this chapter on interviewing techniques has been compiled as a guide for you to follow. You may alter it to fit the particular needs of your department. We have attempted to present this information in an easily readable style. We hope it is helpful to you in the performance of your duties.

The material presented in this chapter need not be limited to employment selections; its basic principles can be used for counseling interviews, routine administrative interviews regarding transfers, promotions, performance, and so on. Each interview has specific objectives, and you should be able to modify these principles somewhat to attain your objectives.

The fundamental importance of sound interviewing techniques cannot be overemphasized. If your selections are good, the hospital will profit by having productive workers, low turnover, stability, punctuality, and overall high esprit de corps. With unwise selections, all results swing in the opposite direction. One needs to protect the interests of both institution and applicant with regard to compliance with the letter and spirit of all civil rights guidelines and laws. In addition, for every person it employs and subsequently terminates because of an unwise selection, the institution is responsible for payments in the form of unemployment compensation.

The major cause of unsatisfactory interviewing and selection results is attributed in most instances to the failure of many hospitals to establish a protocol for the selection, interview, and employment processes. Personnel executives and department heads who complain about snags in their present system may have only themselves to blame. If your process is, in fact, a succession of crisis efforts undertaken haphazardly, the unfortunate results can be predicted. A systematic procedure that includes all or some of the following will prove beneficial in eliminating interviewing and selection bottlenecks.

THE SELECTION/INTERVIEW/EMPLOYMENT PROCESS

1. Notify the Personnel Department of the impending vacancy.
2. Maintain a job posting program (giving those already working for the institution an opportunity to apply for promotions or lateral transfers.)
3. The Personnel Department initiates the recruitment process, using applications on file and/or advertisements.
4. A preliminary interview of applicants is conducted by the Personnel Department.
5. The preliminary data and references are reviewed by the personnel staff.
6. An interview is conducted by the department head.
7. A decision is made by the department head to accept or reject the applicant.*
8. The credential and reference checks are completed (if the applicant is accepted).*
9. All applicants are notified (accepted or rejected).
10. A preemployment physical is given.
11. Processing by the personnel staff is completed (including notification of starting date).
12. Orientation information is given about the hospital, the department, and the position, respectively.
13. The applicant starts work.

There are many different uses for the interview, including employment, job analysis, follow-up after placement, exit, vocational counseling, and so on. However, in this chapter we will concentrate on interviewing as it pertains to the selection process for employment.

There are five distinct parts to every interview (described in greater detail later in this chapter).

1. **Building rapport**

    a) Create a friendly, relaxed atmosphere with proper introductions.
    b) Relate to the applicant by showing an interest in him or her.

---

*Depending on circumstances and the applicant's permission, items 7 and 8 may be reversed or done simultaneously.

2. **Gathering information**

    a) Review work history, education, and experiences.
    b) Ask probing questions to get facts.

3. **Giving information**

    a) Answer questions or give information about the hospital, working conditions, and the job.
    b) The interview may have an additional purpose. The person who conducts the interview may be obligated to sell the applicant on the job. At the least, the interviewer may have to serve as the organization's voice, giving the applicant the information needed to understand the position and to decide whether he or she is interested in it. The interview is an important event in the life of the applicant, who usually has more to lose than the employer if the wrong decision is made. It should be shown that the interviewer senses this and wants the applicant to be well served.

4. **Summing up**

    a) Review high points of the interview and invite questions.
    b) Advise the applicant of his or her status; i.e., the applicant either will be considered further or does not fit your qualifications right now (but the application will be kept on file).

5. **Recording the final decision**

Even though interviewers may not tell the applicant exactly why he or she is not being hired, they must keep accurate records that reflect the reasons for their decisions. These notes should show that each candidate was evaluated solely on the basis of his or her ability to do the job.

There are six basic recognized interview methods (or variations).

1. Planned or structured
2. Nondirective or nonstructured
3. Depth
4. Group
5. Stress
6. Quality-guided

The planned interview is one in which the interviewer has prepared in advance a schedule of questions to be asked. This method is most useful when similar information is required from each applicant.

The **nondirective interview** does not follow a preestablished pattern and is most useful in exploring a broad area. It is used by most personnel directors and is widely accepted as the most effective method.

The **depth interview**, not really a distinct method, goes into considerable detail on one particular and important interview subject. It is not normally used in employment interviewing.

The **group interview** examines a number of individuals simultaneously and is seldom used in private employee selection. This method of interviewing is practical for "hiring halls" and is used for short-term or special large-project hiring.

The **stress interview** is not a distinct method per se. It uses some form of pressure to test the applicant's reactions. It should only be used by an experienced person trained in interviewing techniques.

The **quality-guided interview** is a modified version of the planned or structured interview. It is an inventory of quality points, each of which can be graded by degree. This interview method works very well along with the nondirective or nonstructured method. We will elaborate on the quality-guided interview at the end of this chapter.

WHAT THE INTERVIEWER NEEDS

Before we get into the actual techniques of good interviewing, it is appropriate to discuss what factors you, the interviewer, should make use of to conduct a successful interview.

1. You must have a good working knowledge of the job for which you are interviewing applicants.
2. You must be able to make objective decisions that are free from prejudice. The interviewer's efforts must be devoted solely to the interests of the hospital, and personal feelings must be disregarded.
3. The ability to make sound judgments and accurate estimates is necessary.
4. You need the ability to withstand pressure. The interviewer must be especially careful to remain calm "under fire" and must avoid any loss of temper (or even showing that he or she is disturbed), regardless of how provocative circumstances may become.
5. Empathy, the ability to "put yourself in the other person's shoes" (the imaginative projection of one's own sensitivity into another being), is a trait too frequently missing among interviewers.
6. You should use a private place to conduct your interview, which should be done at leisure and free from interruptions.

7. In addition to the factors already listed, you should have the following qualities.
    a) Good appearance, manners, and dress
    b) Warm, outgoing personality
    c) Sincerity
    d) Enthusiasm
    e) Self-confidence
    f) Initiative

THE APPLICATION FOR EMPLOYMENT

Ideally speaking, you possess all the traits previously mentioned and are now ready to interview, evaluate, and select someone to fill a job position in your department. As a general rule, the first step is to have the person fill out an application for employment. However, since you will be conducting the final interview, the candidate will most likely have already completed an application form from the Personnel Department, and you will have this in your possession when the candidate arrives. Remember that the application form should be carefully designed to meet all of the federal and state guidelines that protect the applicant's rights.

In brief, a variety of *elimination factors* may become readily apparent by merely glancing over an application.

1. To begin with, the experience or education of the applicant may be inadequate for whatever opening you may have; that applicant should be placed in the "Thank you for your interest in our hospital—we'll let you know when we have something for you" category.
2. There are too many jobs of short duration. Applicants in this category are risky. Avoid hiring those with poor work-history records and hoping they'll become model employees for you. The chances are that you'll be disillusioned and will only add to your turnover.
3. Unexplained gaps in the applicant's employment record should be thoroughly explored. A surprising amount of useful information may be secured in this manner.
4. Beware of applications that are replete with misspellings, blots, and erasures or that indicate inability to follow simple directions, e.g., writing when asked to print, or not answering questions.
5. The inevitable "wise guys" occasionally reveal themselves by giving facetious answers to questions on the application.

Within the last two years, legislation designed to protect civil liberties has complicated the employer's efforts regarding reference checks. A negative assessment of a worker by his past employer now appears to legally infringe on that worker's right. Reference sources are touchy.

Many hospitals will no longer release information about past employees for fear of litigation. In short, reference checks are becoming more difficult to obtain. Instead of making normal reference checks, many hospitals are simply verifying data such as dates of employment and position held. If the applicant's data are different from the summation data obtained from the former employer, the applicant is asked for an explanation.

Prospective employers should not forgo reference checks altogether. We suggest that reference checks be made by telephone. Assure the person you are calling that you will guarantee absolute confidentiality. Concentrate on any subtle remarks made about the applicant during your phone conversation. What this person doesn't say about a former employee can often tell you a great deal. Be careful yourself about getting involved in a legal action for giving out unfavorable information on either a prospective or former employee. Remember that the hospital may be required to defend your comments and actions in court. Always be mindful that the rating you give should be objective and honest.

If your institution has a Personnel Department, we suggest that the department heads and supervisors rely on them to initiate and finish all reference checks. The Personnel Department can simplify rather than complicate the task of reference checking.

"WE ARE AN EQUAL OPPORTUNITY EMPLOYER"

Federal and state fair employment requirements defined by antidiscrimination laws are quite specific regarding equal opportunity practices.

The law requires you to recruit and select the most capable individual available for each position with no discrimination made between individuals because of color, ancestry, religious creed, age,* citizenship, race or national origin, marital status, sex, or physical or mental handicap (unless related to a bona fide occupational qualification).

During the interview you may not ask about the following items.

Birth certificate, naturalization papers, baptismal records, or photographs
Union sympathies, if any
Military service discharge papers
Languages (other than English) written, read, or spoken
Place of birth
Birthplace of parents, husband, wife, or any other relatives
Membership in clubs, societies, organizations

---

*Age: The Age Discrimination in Employment Act of 1967 prohibits discrimination on the basis of age with respect to individuals who are at least 40 but less than 70 years of age.

Change of name if by court order
Maiden name of married woman
Religion
Age
Race
Citizenship
National origin
Marital status
Sex (regarding refusal to hire someone just because the job has traditionally been done by a female or a male)

It is also a good policy to avoid comments or discussions relative to the following.

- Politics
- Competitors
- Your personal comments about any person, place, job, or occupation

PREJUDICES TO GUARD AGAINST

You must recognize that your judgment about each applicant must be based on a sound analysis of qualifications for the position and not on a multitude of other influences. Payroll dollars are primarily intended to buy *job performance* for the hospital. We have actually encountered rejections of applicants for such reasons as "She doesn't look like a good worker." "He has a weak face." "She doesn't shake hands as if she meant it." "I know his uncle and if he's like him, I don't want him." "She's no good, I can tell by looking at her." "His mother worked here years ago, and she did not get along well with people."

Just as you should guard against personal prejudices, you should also be careful to guard against hiring (or not hiring) someone just because you know the family or because the applicant is related to someone in the hospital.

INTERVIEWING—GENERAL COMMENTS

Employment interviewing is a skill that needs to be developed. Its goal is specific—employee selection for production, with permanence and adjustability to the hospital. As you screen applicants, you must think constantly of the degree to which the applicant will fit into the hospital picture—into its care for patients and into its requirements of unusual working hours and conditions.

The interview is an active, strenuous process demanding flexibility, skill, and insight on the part of the interviewer. It is hard work. In every interview, you must do two things simultaneously. The first is to gather data. These data include the applicant's behavior during the interview. The interviewer must note not only what the applicant says or feels but also what is not said, and how he or she reacts and handles the interview. The second and more important thing to do at the same time is to look beneath the surface to uncover the meaning and implications of the applicant's behavior. The most important qualities that one must have to know or to predict these implications are those that require the most skill during interviewing. There is no ready, obvious way to take a reading on attitude, aspiration, dependability, or reasoning, but insight concerning these intangible personal qualities can be gained by the interviewer who knows what to look for and recognizes it when he or she finds it.

THE INTERVIEW PROCESS

Put the applicant at ease
(Building rapport—15% of interview time)
It is of the utmost importance to greet the applicant cordially and to make every effort to relax the person and put him or her at ease. The interviewer is responsible for making this effort. During the first minutes, the interviewer should carry the ball with pleasant, light conversation to give the applicant an opportunity to settle down and muster up confidence. The interview can then start off with questions that the applicant can answer without feeling threatened. Penetrating and complex questions should be saved until later in the interview. A technique we have found very helpful after having cordially greeted the applicant and offered a chair is merely to say, "Tell me about yourself." Most reply, "What would you like to know?" Our answer is, "Anything you think important for me to know."

You should note how each applicant starts his or her presentation —with the last job, education, family, plans for the future, or whatever strikes them as primarily important. This unstructured interview method can be extremely illuminating if properly handled, and the applicants will reveal far more of themselves than they expected. Relax and listen; you want to find out about the applicant and the presentation is usually a crucial evaluation point.

Avoid revealing your reactions. Care should be used to avoid showing particular approval or disapproval of what is said to you. Applicants will react to what you say, your manner, and your facial expressions, and they will strive to say whatever they think will gain your approval. A good "poker face" is a real asset in interviewing (but don't go overboard). Some are of the opinion that writing on a form while interviewing makes the interviewee self-conscious and ill at ease. It is best to avoid excessive writing while the person is present. Detailed notes should be made as soon as the interview is over.

Ask probing questions to get facts
(Gathering information – 55% of interview time)

After the applicant stops talking, which some do quite rapidly, certain brief but probing questions must be posed. Avoid asking questions that can be answered with either a yes or no.

"What was a typical day on your previous job like?"
"If you had the authority to change things at your last position, what would you have done first?"
"What does success mean to you?"
"Should you get this job, how will you expect the hospital to assist you in your work?"
"What were the contributing factors that led you to become a (nurse) (aide) (cook)?"
"What are your thoughts on weekend or holiday work?"
"What was your favorite subject in school?"
"What are your plans for the future?"

A group of three or four questions built around the job description for any one job may be of help to the interviewer in determining the actual job knowledge of the applicant. If an experienced worker is sought, he or she should be familiar with methods and terms common to the profession or work category.

Orderly or aide
"How do you transfer a patient from a stretcher to a bed?"
"In what ways can the patient's temperature be taken?"

Laundry worker
"What part of a shirt do you iron first?"
"How do you iron a coat sleeve?"

Nurse
"When do you record medications administered to a patient, before or after the administration?"
"Who administered the IV's at your last place of employment?"

The able interviewer listens actively, having the ability to interpret and understand what the applicant says. If passive listening was enough, the interviewer could be eliminated and the applicant could talk into a tape recorder. The good interviewer does little talking, but what talking he or she does is purposeful and sensitive. The interviewer must remember that the purpose is to elicit responses from the applicant that will provide the insight needed for the hiring decision. The applicant should be induced to talk freely. Too many interviewers talk too much; the wise ones offer only a few key remarks calculated to prompt the responses sought.

Observations in interviewing are part of the information-gathering routine. A good deal can be learned by observation. With a few glances, you should be able to assess the following accurately.

- General appearance
- Grooming habits
- Alertness and promptness of response
- Use of English
- Ease in conversation
- General courtesy or manners

Give the applicant a detailed picture of the job
(Giving information—15% of interview time)

- General nature of the work and a review of the job description
- Hours and days of work
- Holiday coverage
- Weekend coverage
- Attendance requirements
- Uniform requirements
- Rest periods
- Tour of the work area and the department, if possible

The Personnel Department will most likely have covered the following items during the preliminary interview. However, if you wish to review these items again with the applicant, feel free to do so, but be sure you are completely familiar with them.

- Probable beginning salary
- Frequency of salary increments
- Pay schedule
- Benefits (holidays, vacation, insurance, etc.)
- Preemployment physical
- Orientation schedule

Terminate the interview
(Summing up—15% of interview time)

There is a public-relations aspect of interviewing which is almost as important as hiring. Even rejecting applicants is an art; you must expend every effort to make them feel that they have been treated with courtesy and consideration while letting them know where they stand.

Always remember, your paths may cross again. Perhaps the organization is unable to hire these applicants at this time, but it may consider them again in the future. A positive interview will leave them more ready and willing future candidates. They may also return as patients, or be employed by organizations that do business with you or your institution. It will not hurt you a bit to keep in the back of your head the thought that someday an applicant may be your supervisor. Does the interview deal with the applicant in such a way that it lays sound groundwork for that eventuality?

The close of the interview should be carefully planned. It should be done in a friendly manner, with avoidance of any antagonizing comments. If the individual is clearly not qualified for the job, it is best to tell him or her something like "We do not have anything to fit your qualifications right now. We will hold your application and call you if anything develops. Thank you for coming in." Another closing frequently used is "We are still seeing other applicants for this position. We will be sure to get in touch with you within a week or so. Thanks for coming in to see us."

It happens occasionally that an applicant does not budge as you make what you believe to be your "dismissal speech." In that event, a simple but usually effective technique is to rise and head for the door; most people will rise and walk with you. If somewhat sterner measures are in order, should the applicant fail to respond to your rising, try "I wish I could spend more time with you, but I'm late for a meeting and I must leave now." If that does not work, you have a problem; call the Personnel Director, who should then join you.

INTERVIEWING AN APPLICANT FOR AN EXECUTIVE OR SUPERVISORY POSITION

An applicant who asks questions during an interview shows an interest in the job and the institution and also gives the interviewer a better idea of whether the job is right for the applicant. It is not only what the applicant asks that is important, but how and when he or she asks it. The following guidelines have been prepared to assist you in evaluating an applicant for an executive or supervisory position.

If an applicant for an executive or supervisory position asks about any of the following four items before all others during the first interview, the interviewer should be cautious about finalizing employment commitments.

- Salary—the job should be the most important subject. Salary (assuming basic adequacy) should only be mentioned after most of the other concerns about the job have been clarified.
- Salary increases—closely related to the salary syndrome. A more acceptable question for the applicant to ask is, "How long would it be before my work is reviewed?"

- Promotion—you are looking for someone to fill current job needs. You are not trying to discourage mobility; however, you need some assurance that the applicant is not going to use the position as a mere "stepping stone."
- Expenses—travel expenses related to the interview appointment, expense accounts related to the job, and relocation expenses should not overly concern the applicant, unless financial hardship actually exists.

During their first interview, the most favorable applicants should ask most of the following questions, listed in order of importance.

1. Questions that show an interest in the institution
2. Questions about what the responsibilities will be
3. Requirements of the job
4. The location of the job and department in the organizational structure
5. The relationship of the work to that of others and vice versa
6. Questions on the history of the job (incumbents, new position, etc.)
7. Questions related to accountability—to how many people the applicant will be answerable
8. Number of employees to be supervised
9. Degree of autonomy
10. Questions about benefits—medical and educational policies, insurance, pension plans
11. What the hours and vacation time are and which holidays are provided
12. Questions related to salary, travel expenses, relocation expenses

WHAT TO LOOK FOR IN A RESUME

Most important Presence of an address; work experience; college degree, major, and grades in that subject; job goals; date available for work; career objectives; length of time previous jobs were held; spouse's willingness to relocate; health status and any physical limitations (if applicable); job location and travel limitations; acceptable salary; college minor

Less important Years degrees received; overall grade average; awards and scholarships; grades in college minor; offices in professional organizations; name of college; class standing; how much of the money for college expenses was earned; names of references

Unimportant Birth date or age; honorary societies; offices in social organizations; student body offices; hobbies; marital status; college transcript; height and weight; number of children; spouse's occupation or educational level; photograph; religion; personal data on parents

Look for a one-page, typed cover letter that states the job being applied for, why he or she is seeking that particular job, a statement on any current job and career objectives, and an indication that the applicant knows something about the organization. Not essential in the cover letter is who referred the applicant, statements regarding the confidentiality of the application, or references.

Avoid considering resumes that:

- are poorly written, sloppy, or on dirty or stained stationery.
- appear to have been mass produced.
- are addressed improperly (e.g., "Dear Sir or Madam"; "To Whom it may concern") or that have no cover letter.
- are loaded with trivia.
- lack discretion, i.e., critical of former employers, fellow employees, and so on.

A prompt, definitive reply to all resumes received is strongly recommended.

SUGGESTIONS FOR USING THE GUIDED INTERVIEW INVENTORY

The Guided Interview Inventory (Exhibit 11-1) is a list of quality points, each of which can be graded either superior, good, fair, or poor. These quality points are each known to be important considerations. Therefore, a favorable combination of these factors should be present before an applicant is worthy of serious consideration.

During the interviewing discussion, as each quality point and its accompanying factors are explored to a degree sufficient for evaluation, a check mark is placed in that column most closely describing the applicant's degree of acceptability. This process is followed for each of the eighteen items covered. For example, if the applicant makes an unusually fine initial impression, a check mark should be placed in the "Superior" column. Also, any comments qualifying or modifying a rating should be made under "Remarks" on the back of the form. To obtain a true overall appraisal of the applicant's suitability for consideration, each point should be viewed by itself, and no overall rating should be made until a definite impression is gained.

A composite evaluation can best be made by totaling all impressions using the following scoring instructions.

- For each rating of superior, the score of that quality point is 3.
- For each rating of good, the score is 2.
- For each rating of fair, the score is 1.
- No positive score (0) is given for any poor rating.

EXHIBIT 11-1

GUIDED INTERVIEW INVENTORY

	FACTORS TO CONSIDER	SUPERIOR	GOOD	FAIR	POOR	SCORE
1.	GENERAL APPEARANCE	Impression created by dress, grooming, and personal hygiene				
2.	QUALIFICATIONS FOR JOB	Degree of hospital experience of applicant				
a)	EDUCATION	Whether commensurate with job requirements; over- or underqualified				
b)	EMPATHY	Potential contribution to the hospital's objective of maintaining a caring environment				
c)	EXPERIENCE	Job success				
3.	AVAILABILITY REGARDING HOURS OF WORK	Availability for shift work, weekends, holidays				
4.	APPEARANCE OF APPLICATION FORM	Handwriting, completeness, accuracy				

Exhibit 11-1 (continued)

	FACTORS TO CONSIDER	SUPERIOR	GOOD	FAIR	POOR	SCORE
5.	CONVERSATIONAL ABILITY	Ability to express himself or herself					
6.	ATTITUDES	Sense of fairness and loyalty					
7.	PERSUASIVENESS	Enthusiasm; interest in getting the job; self-confidence					
8.	ALERTNESS	Reactions to questions; quickness in grasping the point being discussed					
9.	AMBITION	Aims and goals; desire to succeed; drive					
10.	INTERESTS	Leadership tendencies; interest in the institution					
11.	SALARY/WAGES	Beginning salary rate not less than needs or previous earnings					
12.	STABILITY	Number of jobs and reasons for changes					

Exhibit 11-1 (continued)

	FACTORS TO CONSIDER	SUPERIOR	GOOD	FAIR	POOR	SCORE
13.	MOTIVATION	The need to feel secure through own efforts					
14.	MATURITY	Levelheadedness; belief in hard work; sound judgment					
15.	POTENTIAL	Chances of success and potential for advancement					
	TOTAL SCORE					

The scores are added at the bottom and can be interpreted using the following table.

Score	Overall rating
42 to 54	Superior
29 to 41	Good
16 to 28	Fair
0 to 15	Poor

Normally only those whose final grading corresponds to "Good" or better should be considered as favorable employment risks. However, individual judgment remains the crux of the entire hiring procedure. "Poor" ratings in vital areas along with an otherwise high score would naturally be sufficient cause for elimination. It is important to analyze how good the favorable aspects are in relation to how bad the disadvantages may be. The Guided Interview Inventory serves as a reminder of the factors you will want to weigh in passing overall judgment on each applicant. Obviously qualified or unqualified applicants cause no decision problems, but those who may be borderline in some areas deserve your careful consideration.

When you decide to employ an applicant, write a brief statement describing your overall judgment and what prompted you to decide in his or her favor. You may also want to comment on your new employee's strong points as well as those that could be improved through training and supervision.

SUMMARY

Basic do's and don'ts of interviewing

DO:
1. use a quiet, comfortable place.
2. put the applicant at ease.
3. be interested in the person as well as the job.
4. outline clearly the requirements of the job.
5. explain fully the conditions of employment.
6. encourage the applicant to ask questions; give clear answers.
7. listen; let the applicant talk freely.
8. be natural; use a conversational tone.
9. guide the interview.
10. talk about salary, benefits, promotions, and opportunities.
11. know when and how to close the interview.
12. announce your decision or explain your next step.

DON'T:
1. keep the applicant waiting.

2. build false hopes.
3. oversell the job.
4. interrupt the applicant or the interview.
5. rush through the interview.
6. repeat questions already answered on the application or resume.
7. develop a "canned" interview approach.
8. give opinions.
9. pry into the applicant's personal life needlessly.
10. prejudge and reflect prejudices.
11. use a phony excuse for turning the applicant down.
12. send the applicant away with negative feelings about you or the institution.

Other helpful suggestions to consider

1. Don't be impressed because the applicant graduated from a prestigious college or university. There are good universities and colleges at which total costs are less than at some of the more glamorous ones; their graduates are frequently overlooked in the selection process.
2. Top-notch men and women in any line of work are seldom unemployed.
3. An indisputable fact of life is that the executive who has never been unemployed and has had a very successful career may not project a favorable first impression.
4. Look beyond the resume. *Never* hire a person on resume content alone; check the information.

Is the job right for the applicant?

For a successful placement, a "yes" answer to all five items is a must.

1. *A chance to use skills* A job that challenges ingenuity or skill gives a sense of accomplishment.
2. *A feeling that the work is useful* If an employee cannot see the point of labor, self-esteem suffers, which is then reflected in job performance.
3. *An opportunity to participate in decisions* Too much supervision or overly authoritarian direction often creates friction on the job.
4. *A sense of security* Though a job may be just about ideal, an employee will not be happy in it for long if there is a fear that it may be yanked away at any time.
5. *Compensation that is adequate* Money should not provide the main motivation, yet it should not be obviously inappropriate to the individual's personal circumstances.

the earned-time concept

A relatively new approach to granting paid leave combines earned benefits such as vacation, holiday, and sick days into one aggregate of days. More than one term has been used to describe this approach. In this chapter it will be referred to as earned time. The fundamental difference between an earned-time program and the traditional type is that the former combines several types of paid leave and is administered as a single program or benefit instead of several separate ones. For example, an employee who was traditionally entitled to ten days of vacation, nine holidays, and five days of sick time has, under a consolidated earned-time program, 24 days to use any way the employee sees fit.

The purpose of this chapter as it relates to payroll costs is (1) to explain the concept combining various benefits into one program, and (2) to describe the various advantages and disadvantages of such a program.

CONSOLIDATING EMPLOYEE BENEFITS

The general trend of employee benefits, particularly during the 1960s, can be summarized in one word: *more*. During this period, benefits for hospital workers advanced more rapidly than in many other nonmanufacturing industries. This was a catching-up period for hospitals. By 1970 the growth rates of the traditional types of employee benefits had leveled off somewhat, but new benefits have undergone rigorous development. The fastest-growing benefits have been those related to various insurance programs, coverage for which increased 264 percent in all industries since 1967.

Expenditures for employee benefit programs are increasing, and the trend is toward more (or in some instances, complete) employer financing of premium payments and self-insurance. Because the concept is rather new, there are no standardized specifications for such a program. An institution interested in developing a program may consider combining all types of paid leave. On the other hand, it may elect to combine only two, such as vacation and holidays. Factors that would influence program design include (1) the general philosophy of the hospital regarding employee benefits, (2) the institution's financial strength, (3) the degree of dissatisfaction with, or the perceived inequities of, the present program, and (4) prevalent community policies.

In setting up guidelines for an earned-time program, four different areas should be considered: vacation, sick leave (accumulated, taken, and paid), holidays, and miscellaneous benefits such as military and bereavement leave and jury duty.

It is vitally important to determine the amount of time each employee is actually receiving under the traditional (present) program and then convert this to the new program. Data for a period of 12 to 24 months should be used to determine the actual amount each employee has received. Averages are then calculated for sick time, holidays, and miscellaneous time. Since accrued vacation days usually increase based on years of service, earned-time benefits should reflect higher total days for those employees.

Exhibit 12–1 depicts a typical earned-time plan. It shows accumulation for full-time employees only. Prorated accruals should be given to all part-time employees.

ADVANTAGES AND DISADVANTAGES

In 1974 a study was undertaken to obtain information from hospitals that had implemented earned-time programs. Participants were asked to express their opinions regarding advantages and disadvantages of the earned-time program.

The following list illustrates the results of that survey. Advantages and disadvantages are listed by order of frequency.

Advantages

1. Allows the organization to compete more successfully for employees
2. Enhances employee morale
3. Provides better employer–employee relationship
4. Easier to administer benefits as one program rather than many
5. Generates employee loyalty
6. Allows employees to select their own holidays
7. Does not reward those who abuse short-term sick leave or penalize those who don't
8. Discourages the use of sick leave or unexcused absences
9. Increases productivity

Disadvantages

1. Creates a relatively high financial cost
2. Creates staffing and scheduling problems
3. Difficult for some employees to grasp the concept; they still think in terms of sick days, holidays, etc.
4. Employees often use entire allowance too early in the year
5. Encourages excessive absenteeism
6. Difficult to obtain union acceptance of the approach

The most frequently mentioned advantage was that of recruitment, while the most frequently mentioned disadvantage was the relatively high financial cost.

Experience has shown that an earned-time program does result in an increase in total paid days, particularly if provisions are made for occurrences such as extended illnesses.

EXHIBIT 12–1

EARNED-TIME ACCUMULATION PLAN — FULL-TIME EMPLOYEES

	UNDER 5 YEARS	5 YEARS BUT LESS THAN 10 YEARS	10 YEARS AND OVER
VACATION	10 days	15 days	20 days
HOLIDAYS	9 days	9 days	9 days
AVERAGE SICK LEAVE	5 days	5 days	5 days
TOTAL ANNUAL PAID LEAVE	24 days	29 days	34 days

YEARS OF SERVICE	HOURS ACCUMULATED EACH PAY PERIOD
Less than 5 years	3.7 hours
5 years but less than 10 years	4.5 hours
10 years and over	5.2 hours

measurement and analysis of absenteeism and tardiness

Excessive absenteeism, a crippling problem in any institution, is an even greater problem in a health care institution, because it jeopardizes the quality of patient care in addition to imposing a financial burden on the institution. Estimates based on national insurance claims indicate that 300 million man-days are lost each year to certified illnesses alone. Volumes of available literature discuss the causes of absenteeism and suggest methods for controlling it. However, any program to control absenteeism must be tailor-made. It should be based on the characteristics of a specific institution and its employees, because rates of absenteeism vary from one institution to another. Among the reasons for varying rates are: the composition of the work force, including the ratio of part-time to full-time and female to male employees; the type of working environment; and job satisfaction.

The purpose of this chapter is to explain a simple methodology that hospitals can use to determine rates of absenteeism (including excessive absenteeism). In addition, we will also explore various reasons for absenteeism. Armed with this knowledge, supervisors can better direct their efforts toward controlling abuses (see Chapter 14).

A high absence rate means both a high cost for any given hospital and also that workers simply cannot perform as effectively as they can when the rate is low. Managers begin to understand the astounding cost of absenteeism when they realize that, for example, a 4 percent absence rate means that in 25 years the entire work force was absent for a whole year! It is very important to recognize that by using relatively simple, inexpensive measures, absenteeism can be cut as low as possible, thus saving a major proportion of existing productivity otherwise lost to absenteeism, without requiring compensatory actions such as stringent economy moves, greater industrial achievement, or expensive advertising and selling campaigns.

The few employees causing most absences may be difficult to spot without analysis of accurate data. Therefore, in order to determine absenteeism and tardiness, it is absolutely essential that exact and complete records be maintained.

A MEASUREMENT SYSTEM

There is perhaps no other benefit that creates as much concern for both the employer and the employee as the sick leave benefit program. Unfortunately, managers have attempted to present an expanded concept of benefit with a tightened system of control so that on one hand, the employee assumes a good benefit, and on the other hand, receives a minimum value from the benefit. The position of employees, established primarily through collective bargaining demands, has been to concentrate on sick leave as an actual benefit of so many days per year. The management's position is that sick leave is comparable to unilateral insurance provided by the employer for the purpose of maintaining an employee's wage when he or she is sick and unable to work. Based on the premise that one does not get a rebate on hospitalization or life or disability insurance under normal conditions, it is felt that the employee should not benefit from sick leave when not sick. Thus employees may claim sickness that, in effect, aggravates the absentee problem and becomes an added and unnecessary expense to the sick leave benefit program.

A primary difficulty has been managers attempting to use sick leave as some form of attendance-control system rather than separating attendance control from the sick leave benefit. The move toward earned-time benefit programs has established the principle that employees be granted so many days per year, accumulated at a certain rate per month. These days can be taken as vacation days, holidays, sick days, or whatever type of day the employee wants. The management controls the maximum amount of time, but the employee determines the use of this time.

Attendance evaluation can be based on a mathematical formula that multiplies the frequency of absence by the number of days of absence in the preceding 12-month period; the product is then used as a guide to possible disciplinary action. For example, if an employee is absent twice during the year, for 2 days the first time and 4 days the second, there is a frequency of 2 and a number of days of 6. By multiplying 2 by 6, the product of 12 is obtained as an absence rate. Similarly, another employee might be absent 1 day each time for 6 times during the same 12-month period. This results in a frequency of 6×6 for a product of 36. An evaluation scale for possible action is given by four ranges: a product of 18 or less—no problem; 19 through 28—a pending problem requiring counseling; 29 through 36—a serious problem requiring minor discipline; 37 and above—a very serious problem requiring severe discipline, possible suspension, or even discharge.

Another acceptable though less precise evaluation formula is to determine 3.5 percent of the employee's annual work time; the number of days absent per year should not exceed this figure. For example, Helen is a full-time employee who theoretically works 40 hours per week for 52 weeks per year, or 2080 hours per year. When her vacation time of 80 hours and holiday time of 72 hours are subtracted, the final total is 1928 hours of actual work time per year. The figure of $8\frac{1}{2}$ days ($67\frac{1}{2}$ hours) is then obtained by calculating 3.5 percent of 1928; Helen's days absent should, therefore, certainly not be any more than 9.

THE ANALYSIS OF ABSENTEEISM AND TARDINESS

IDENTIFYING ABSENTEES

Chronic absentees are frequently malcontents who either may not have had the opportunity to mature properly or have not yet learned that happiness and satisfaction on the job are derived largely from conscientious work performed to the best of one's ability. Since the supervisor acts as the absentee's counselor, it is necessary for him or her to become completely familiar with the underlying causes of absenteeism in order to be properly prepared to handle absentees in a poised, professional manner.

UNDERLYING CAUSES OF ABSENTEEISM

A lack of social pressure   Sociologists demonstrate social pressures with the classic example of a small community where people traditionally and faithfully go to church. The church absentee is visited, the cause investigated, and the positive help (or negative gossip) creates pressure to return. In contrast, today many people do not stay in one community social group long enough to establish deep roots and to feel social pressures. Positive social pressure is almost absent today, and family pressure is also decreasing. Much of what now remains is negative criticism. Such negative pressure is of little value without strong, positive leadership also being present in the home to help children identify with positive attributes. However, positive attributes are too easily overshadowed by negative attitudes that cast a pall on the home environment. Everything possible must be done to help employees from inadequate homes adjust to their own environment and become rehabilitated.

Today the individual and his or her personal rights and concerns often seem more important, and group interests are for the most part secondary. Even in some sports, team effort is gradually giving way to special attention to key individuals whose presence or absence is credited with victory or defeat. Similarly, superstars in industry have staggering motivating pressures, but those in less glamorous positions require special motivation to keep on the job faithfully for less glory and less pay in their supporting roles.

The health team has been defined as the physician, the patient, and the associated health professionals. To that group must be added the co-worker, the supervisor, and the family, so that with each case a new ad hoc team is formed and tailored to the specific needs of that case. Among the goals of the health team should be to make every employee feel wanted by means of positive efforts and to make every reasonable effort toward rehabilitation.

A changing work force   Recently, both government and industry have been giving more jobs to those who would otherwise be marginally unemployable or who are occupationally inadequate to some degree. The absence rate of unemployables will always be higher than the rate of better-adjusted employees. Many older workers give the impression of having better physical health and resistance to illness as well as greater emotional stamina, since their absences are fewer than those of younger workers. The attitude of getting to work in spite of borderline feelings or symptoms of indisposition paradoxically seems to be a characteristic of older workers, who experience those negative feelings more often, rather than of their younger, more buoyant co-workers.

However, a high degree of constitutional strength is seldom seen in those who have a family history of unemployment, lack of education, and a lack of proper medical attention. The emotional consequences of these handicaps are well known, and some employees from this category feel secure knowing they can make about the same income from charity, unemployment, or welfare payments as they can by actually working. This attitude is partially due to the diminishing of the social stigma attached to the jobless. This group is particularly hard to inspire with company loyalty and job devotion. The problems they present are basically related to their handicaps and immaturity.

Immaturity   Absenteeism can often be correlated with the size of an emotionally immature employee's medical file, which may have hundreds of entries. The tragic tales of these absentees are countless variations on the main theme: immaturity. If immaturity could be eradicated, most "person" problems would be eliminated, leaving much more time for everyone to concentrate on solving "thing" problems.

The Menninger[1] criteria for maturity are (1) having the ability to deal constructively with reality, (2) having the capacity to adapt to change, (3) having relative freedom from symptoms that are produced by tensions and anxieties, (4) having the capacity to find more satisfaction in giving than in receiving, (5) having the capacity to relate to other people in a consistent manner, with mutual satisfaction and helpfulness, (6) having the capacity to redirect one's instinctive hostile energy into creative and constructive outlets, and (7) having the capacity to love.

For supervisors to avoid overreacting while being objective, tolerant, helpful, and understanding, it must be remembered that absentees have simply had insufficient examples to follow and few opportunities to become mature.

An overemphasis on health   While the main purpose of medicine is to promote health, overemphasis on health in the mass media frequently results in hypochondria. The hypochondriac employee may erroneously believe that previous physicians who treated him were wrong in their diagnoses, and he may abuse the patient–doctor relationship repeatedly until mutual disenchantment sets up a cycle of changing doctors. This

---

[1] Karl A. Menninger, noted American psychiatrist, is the founder of the Menninger Foundation, Topeka, Kansas.

pattern infringes on work time, and absences increase without health improvement. Hypochondriacs must be taught to distinguish between serious and minor symptoms, but this obviously is no easy undertaking.

Outside distraction Supervisors must be aware of the reasons for chronic tardiness in employees. Moonlighting, late-night TV watching, and other outside activities that infringe on rest are bound to lessen the normal drive to get out of bed in the morning and get to work on time. Being chronically tired in the morning, the employee uses a variety of imaginary illnesses as excuses when explaining tardiness to the supervisor or company physician. It takes great patience and understanding to deal with this situation, because although the employee is responsible for the fatigue, he or she really does not feel well.

This behavior often starts in school and can be checked before hiring by examining absence and tardiness records. Actually, it is not laziness but rather a form of disorganized living. Many disorganized people have a tendency toward frequent tardiness. Since they are allowed so many sick days per year, they consciously or unconsciously stretch their tardiness into an absence. This activity is an attempt to change the embarrassing situation of tardiness into the "legitimate" one of absence.

Poor motivation Up to a point, it is not unreasonable to expect that time off the job should be spent getting recharged for better work performance. After all, work consumes a large part of every normal person's daily time. But what if work is not really a large part of the employee's daily time? What if he or she is dissatisfied with the job?

There are many reasons for dissatisfaction, of course, and most of them seriously impair motivation. For example, if anticipated opportunities for worthwhile achievement or meaningful progress are either delayed or eliminated, the individual becomes touchy and starts to find fault with the employer.

On the other hand, the employee who is given a challenging job with the possibility of growth, achievement, and advancement to satisfy the need for recognition will enjoy coming to work and performing to the best of his or her ability. The supervisor ordinarily provides these conditions and knows the ways to maintain motivation, occasionally requesting assistance with health problems from the physician. The physician must then be capable of accepting the referral from the supervisor and must also have a good understanding of people to communicate effectively with employees at all levels. Effective communications are needed especially with the front-line supervisors, who most often represent the management to the employees.

Having discussed some general environmental and social elements in the absentee problem, we now turn to specific medical problem areas that are of concern to the company. Of these, psychiatric disorders are responsible for nearly all correctable absenteeism.

Alcoholism Alcoholism is an age-old social, physical, and environmental problem, but today it is generally considered as a psychiatric one. In any case, it is estimated to cause, on average, 3 percent of industrial absenteeism. By 1976, over 60 percent of the top 100 companies in the "Fortune 500" had alcoholism rehabilitation programs.

Actually, mental problems may not be the underlying cause of alcoholism. Nonalcoholics apparently often have the same mental problems as alcoholics. Nevertheless, alcoholism creates "lost weekends," increases marital flareups, destroys physical health, brings financial crisis, and causes criminal and other antisocial behavior. All of this sooner or later catches up with the employee, who has to lose work time because he or she is caught in a vicious, downward spiral.

Nonmedical drug problems The current explosion of nonmedical drug use has again become a true personnel problem, as was the case with morphine addiction after the Civil War, which was aptly called the "soldier's disease." Today it is people of all age groups and from varied social backgrounds coming into the labor market who range in drug use from total abstainers to hard-core addicts. A much greater number of people of all ages are now becoming involved in the use of drugs. A new awareness of this hazard has resulted in both government and private groups working toward the proper solution of this continuing problem. Nevertheless, nonmedical drug abuse is a growing cause of absenteeism, and it will require expert management to prevent drug abuse from someday superseding alcoholism as a major cause of absenteeism in this country.

Other emotional problems The emotionally healthy person has adequate mechanisms for controlling hostility, anxiety, and guilt. This ability comes almost exclusively from the home, where children identify with their parents and imitate them consciously and subconsciously. But if parents do not or cannot provide reassuring and edifying adult behavior, the child rarely succeeds in learning to handle emotions properly, unless other wholesome and strongly influential adult contacts are at hand. Narcissistic or other self-centered behavior disorders caused by parental failings are, in turn, primarily responsible for the failure to respect appointments and work hours.

Those who enjoy their work seldom neglect it, but emotionally troubled employees have difficulty enjoying anything. By studying their psychiatric backgrounds, the supervisor and the company physician usually find the causes of chronic absentees' defective habits.

Physical illness   The primary medical causes of absenteeism are psychiatric, but some physical causes are so frequent that they deserve mention: the common cold, migraine headaches, flu, menstrual disturbances, diarrhea, ankle sprains, and back injuries. These are largely unpreventable, but a sound "home-background" philosophy and good medical support usually keep them from becoming major causes of absenteeism.

The control of physical problems related to serious chronic physical disabilities is a problem of rehabilitative medicine. The absences these problems bring about are unpreventable but are ordinarily not detrimental to work habits. The handicapped worker usually has a commendable attendance record, but serious chronic diseases such as severe diabetes may cause higher than average absence rates.

controlling absenteeism and tardiness

Controlling absenteeism is a one-to-one situation in that the supervisor and the employee face each other and candidly discuss attendance. The effective supervisor can keep absenteeism at an acceptable level. In institutions where absenteeism is a problem it is up to the front-line supervisor to correct it. It is human nature to try to get away with doing things that shouldn't be done. That same trait is shown by absentee employees.

If the potential absentee knows that he or she will be questioned on returning to work, the employee will have a tendency to avoid that confrontation and stay away from work only when it is absolutely necessary. One should not go overboard in questioning absentee reasons, because employees are going to be absent once in a while for perfectly valid reasons. However, occasional legitimate absences should be minimal, and the skilled supervisor should be able to distinguish between legitimate and illegitimate absences. Some supervisors advocate attendance bonuses as a sure way of controlling absenteeism. These bonuses come in various sizes and shapes. Some hospitals claim they work; if they do, it is infrequent. In a majority of situations, employees who receive bonuses are the same employees who would keep their record above reproach anyway. Bonuses cost money, and paying bonuses for good attendance is a form of fiscal irresponsibility.

There are two basic approaches in dealing with the problem of tardiness. The first is to confront the guilty employees each time they are late and remind them of the proper starting time. The second is to remind them each day just before the end of the work day of your anticipation that tomorrow they will be on time. If the situation does not improve, it is time to begin a series of written warnings. Occasional tardiness is easier to tolerate than habitual lateness. The chronic latecomer represents a problem similar to that of the employee who abuses attendance requirements. And remember, the supervisor has to set a good example by being on time—employees expect to see the supervisor on the job when they arrive. There are advocates who declare that pay docking is the panacea for tardiness. Unfortunately, what this does is give the employee a legitimate reason for tardiness: "Why should you complain if I'm late; I'm not getting paid for the time."

The best method for controlling absenteeism and tardiness is prevention. Prevention can only be accomplished by treating each incident seriously, keeping accurate attendance records, and properly advising or reminding employees of your attendance expectations.

As a matter of institutional policy the control of absenteeism must be promulgated as a serious endeavor. This endeavor requires the complete understanding and support of every supervisor in every department if it is to be realized. All supervisory personnel must be made aware that the control of absenteeism is their direct responsibility and will require the best relationships between themselves and their employees.

Top management should establish attendance policies and the supervisory responsibilities and accountabilities necessary for controlling absenteeism. The institution's attendance policy should state:

"Each employee was hired as a person important and necessary to the fulfillment of the objectives and obligations of the institution, and, therefore, each person is needed every day that he or she is supposed to be on the job. If this was not true, the employee would surely not have been hired by the institution.

Sick leave is offered by the institution only for illness emergencies that might otherwise result in poor or hazardous work performance or create an unexpected financial burden for employees. All employees, including managers, must aim for perfect attendance records. Perfect attendance can be achieved by living and working safely at all times whether at home or at work, taking timely preventive measures against sickness and injury, and never allowing minor illnesses or other minor problems to prevent work attendance at the proper time.

The institution is forced to recognize all absences or tardiness as significantly detrimental in that it weakens the institution's ability to achieve its goals, services, and productivity. No one is exempted from the need to strive for perfect attendance, and, therefore, good attendance is one of the most important criteria for continued employment. In fairness to employees who exert maximum effort to maintain perfect attendance records, the institution must terminate employees who do not comply with its attendance policy . . . ."

The supervisor is directly responsible for the promotion of good attendance. Most employees will respond positively to demonstrations of appreciation and recognition of their excellent attendance. This recognition may be shown by verbal commendations, by letter, or by certificates of appreciation from the management.

For employees with chronic absence or tardiness problems, the supervisor must candidly discuss this record with the employee and firmly state that the institution cannot afford to tolerate a continued pattern of absenteeism or tardiness. The supervisor should use a calendar-type attendance form that accurately depicts the quantity of and the reasons for absences or tardiness. When dealing with a true, chronic absentee, it is essential for the supervisor to closely monitor all types of absences. This is necessary because many chronic absentees have developed rather sophisticated methods for finding legitimate ways of getting out of work that show up as excessive "excused" absences.

CONTROLLING ABSENCE BY SUPERVISORY ACTION

The disciplinary action taken may be divided into several stages.

THE FIRST ABSENCE

Initially the supervisor should record the absence and check with the employee early on the first day of return regarding the reason for the absence. This information should be recorded both on the calendar attendance records and on the Written Warning form (see Chapter 9). If the absence was for medical reasons, it may be necessary at this stage to refer the employee to the Personnel Health Office or to counsel the employee regarding your attendance expectations. During the interview, it is important to review the institution's policy regarding attendance with the employee and to document this discussion on a Report of Counseling Interview form (Exhibit 14-1).

OCCASIONAL RECURRING UNEXCUSED ABSENCES

If absenteeism continues, the employee should be clearly warned that his or her position and even employment are now at stake if unexcused absences occur again. This should be fully documented on the Written Warning form, including the remarks of the employee.

THE FINAL WARNING

If absenteeism continues, the supervisor is obliged to inform the employee that this is the last chance before termination of employment. This last warning should be put in writing by the supervisor.

TERMINATION

If another unexcused absence then occurs, the employee is terminated for excessive absenteeism.

If the supervisor becomes aware of a possible physical or psychiatric problem underlying the absence, the employee should be immediately referred to the Personnel Health Office for rehabilitation at any stage before termination.

The problems of absenteeism and tardiness are frequently legitimate, and each employee has to be handled on an individual basis. The reasons for absenteeism and tardiness are many and varied. Many rea-

EXHIBIT 14-1

REPORT OF COUNSELING INTERVIEW

Employee name _____

Position _____ Department _____

REASON FOR COUNSELING _____

_____

_____

_____

RECOMMENDED ACTION _____

_____

_____

_____

Supervisor signature _____

Employee signature _____

Date _____

sons are unique. The supervisor needs to examine each case on its own merit. Does the absenteeism or tardiness create a work-flow problem for your department? Is it creating poor morale? Can you live with the situation? Do you want or need to correct it? The best way to work toward a solution is with understanding and recognition of the problem (see Chapter 13).

SUMMARY

Absenteeism can be kept to an absolute minimum. However, it requires continuous first-line supervisory attention.

1. The supervisor must be able to convince employees that it is to their advantage to maintain good attendance records.
2. Accurate attendance records that will reveal absence patterns must be maintained.
3. Employees must be questioned about the reasons for absences.
4. Supervisors must never forget to record that an employee was absent on a scheduled work day.
5. New employees must be oriented to attendance expectations.
6. Employees with good attendance records should not be allowed to develop poor habits. Their absences should also be questioned.

15

controlling unemployment and workmen's compensation costs

CONTROLLING UNEMPLOYMENT COSTS

Claims for unemployment compensation usually begin when a former employee files an application at the local Employment Security Office. The employer will then receive a "Request for Separation Information" form. It is extremely important that the employer complete the form accurately and totally. It is useful as well as advantageous to use appropriate language on the form, e.g., if an employee resigned, use the terminology as defined in the law—the employee "voluntarily quit." Or if an employee was discharged for cause, the language for this violation of work rules should again use the terminology set forth in the law—the employee was "discharged for misconduct" and go on to explain the reasons why. Give as much detail as possible on the form, because the deputy's decision to grant or deny benefits is based on the information on this form as well as that supplied by the former employee.

Good, well-documented personnel records are essential. When employees resign, make sure a written resignation form is signed by the employee. If an employee quits and gives no notice (walks off the job), have the employee's supervisor write the facts and submit them to the Personnel Office to be filed in the employee's record.

If an employee is discharged for misconduct, i.e., violation of a hospital work rule, it is essential that the following conditions exist and are documented.

1. There is evidence of progressive discipline—the employee is given a series of oral and written warnings. Be sure the employee has knowledge of the warnings. In fact, it's good practice to have the employee sign the warning and then have a copy placed in his personnel file.
2. The discipline shows due process. The employee has the opportunity to appeal the warning, termination, or whatever.
3. The dismissal itself is completely documented with regard to the circumstances.

The importance of well-documented personnel files cannot be overemphasized, particularly when employees are trying to prove an improper discharge for misconduct. The burden of proof lies with the employer.

Once a deputy has made a decision about the employee's claim to benefits based on the separation information and other data, this initial decision may be appealed to a higher authority (appeals tribunal) by either party. Don't hesitate to appeal any decision if you feel the judgment is not right.

If an effort fails and former employees do collect benefits, this group becomes an excellent source of applicants for current openings.

The Personnel Director can use his or her discretion and offer positions to appropriately qualified former employees.

Offers of suitable employment should be made to employees collecting benefits, even if it involves a different shift. Quite often, employees will refuse work on an undesirable shift. This will, however, result in their disqualification for unemployment benefits.

Unemployment compensation can be controlled. Develop a system to monitor the entire process, from the "request for separation" information to the appeal process. Be careful to check all terminating employees' personnel files for completeness and documentation. Being diligent will have its rewards.

WORKMEN'S COMPENSATION

Although the costs of workmen's compensation are to some degree not controllable by the hospital (i.e., the state setting maximum benefits), there are areas which should be investigated. Many hospitals have had insurance coverage with one company for a number of years. Before renewing with the same firm, an effort should be made each year to shop around and negotiate for better rates. One Pennsylvania hospital reported a $30,000 savings by renegotiating its coverage with a new carrier.

Self-insuring workmen's compensation has been receiving a great deal of attention lately, in which the hospital may assume the risk to a certain dollar amount, with an insurance carrier covering catastrophic losses. Factors to be considered in this type of self-insurance are administrative costs and the cost of assuming training support that is possibly being provided currently by your insurance carrier. Self-insurance of any type does present a problem if the hospital has an insurance carrier who provides several types of coverage in a policy. The carrier may be unwilling to write coverage for other types of risks unless workmen's compensation is also included.

An aggressive safety program with support from your insurance carrier can do much to reduce losses. One individual in the hospital should be designated as a "safety officer" who reviews employee injuries and accidents in an effort to isolate and correct unsafe conditions and practices. For example, employees need periodic reminders on proper lifting techniques. Mandatory attendance at such reminder meetings should be required of all employees who have sustained injuries as a result of lifting activities. A good publicity campaign with positive reinforcement concerning safe conditions and practices is a must.

evaluating
the
performance
of employees

The most demanding and important responsibility that a supervisor has is the task of accurately appraising the performance of employees. Performance appraisal charges supervisors with the challenge of defining the quality of work that is being done under their direct guidance. By virtue of the type of work done in health care institutions, hospital supervisors have far greater responsibilities in the evaluation process than do their counterparts in industry. The job of managing and developing human resources in hospitals has become increasingly complex. Unquestionably, the quality of work in the health care industry will become an even more important issue in the years ahead. Supervisors will also need to deal with new social and individual values in the workplace. The era is ending wherein supervisors could conduct a superficial performance evaluation merely by walking to one of their employees and saying, "You do good work; I'm going to recommend you for a raise."

It has been said that there is nothing to compare with your job to make you believe in yourself. It is common for supervisors to inadvertently create ambivalent feelings between themselves and their employees by failing to recognize the human-relation keys to inner feelings and understanding: appreciation, explanations, listening, and respect. The supervisor's ability to use those human-relation keys will determine his or her skill in the evaluation process.

An effort has been made to present the material in this chapter in a methodical style that will quickly acquaint the reader with the basics of the evaluation process.

The emphasis is on *employee evaluation*, also known as performance evaluation, which in itself is a highly interesting and provocative topic. In management circles and in business literature knowledgeable management people write emphatically, pro and con, on the performance evaluation question. There are as many views on the subject as there are theories on human behavior.

Surveys usually show that most people think the idea of performance appraisal is good. They feel that a person should know where he or she stands. Therefore, supervisors should discuss performance with their employees periodically.

This chapter has been prepared in the hope that it will be of some help to supervisors when they are rating employees. Its contents are by no means exhaustive; in fact, it can be considered a synopsis of the subject of evaluations.

Our main goal is to acquaint supervisors with both the importance and the process of evaluating workers. We have deliberately excluded the types of forms to be used. Our experience indicates that the form by itself is irrelevant to the process. There are several good performance evaluation forms to be found in several business-form catalogs. See also Exhibits 1–1 and 1–2 in Chapter 1.

A DESCRIPTION OF PERFORMANCE EVALUATION

Performance evaluation is a systematic and objective assessment of an employee's performance, and it is important to both the hospital and the employee. Performance evaluation is also all of the following.

1. A *management tool* used to determine the performance level of each employee
2. A *plan* for forming comparable judgments of the various capacities of different individuals
3. A *technique* to focus the attention of both the supervisor and the employee on the work situation
4. An *instrument* used to reduce or eliminate irrelevant traits
5. A *design* to replace haphazard or unsystematic estimates of the employee's performance

PURPOSES OF PERFORMANCE EVALUATIONS

1. To improve performance and morale by praise, encouragement, or constructive criticism
2. To establish performance goals for future evaluations
3. To provide a permanent record of employee performance
4. To provide a predictable and understandable structure in which the supervisor evaluates an employee and discusses performance
5. To assure the employee that his or her contribution is important and that the supervisor is concerned about each employee as an individual
6. To afford the employee an opportunity to discuss his or her performance and any difficulties
7. To hear employee suggestions that may improve methods, performance, or morale
8. To enhance the caring-environment image of the institution

Hospitals need to be keenly interested in satisfactory performance. Just because an applicant has been selected, hired, placed on the job, oriented, and trained is no certainty that he or she will perform as expected. Performance may be adequate, below standard, or even above average. But how do we know? An evaluation serves the very practical function of reviewing the worker's performance in an attempt to answer the question "How well is the employee doing?" It has an important specific purpose, which is to improve performance, though it may also be used for career guidance appraisals, promotion appraisals, transfers, and determining training needs. These latter uses, however, are secondary; the primary purpose is to improve the worker's performance and to acknowledge those whose performance is meritorious. It is unrealistic to expect a single appraisal to achieve every conceivable need. Separate appraisals can be done for different purposes.

Perfection on all levels is something that doubtless will never be found or established in any organization. Hence the use of a tool becomes necessary to assist those who are in need of improvement and to recognize those that are doing a good job. The performance evaluation process is that tool.

BENEFITS OF PERFORMANCE EVALUATIONS

Any enterprise with a well-organized performance evaluation program will derive a considerable number of benefits from it. These benefits follow.

1. The strengths and weaknesses of each employee become part of a permanent record that can be utilized for transfers, promotions, and career guidance.
2. Supervisors are made aware of the differences among their employees.
3. An effective evaluation program develops better supervisors.
4. Training needs become readily ascertainable.
5. The evaluation process serves as a stimulus for individuals to improve.
6. The management becomes better aware of supervisory abilities as a result of checking ratings.
7. The hiring process may be improved by studying correlations between ratings and past selection of new applicants.
8. Patients are better served and the quality of care increases.
9. The institution's image as a humanitarian, caring environment improves and grows.

HOW TO START INFORMAL PERFORMANCE EVALUATION DISCUSSIONS

Impromptu, informal discussions are best. The best time to discuss an employee's work with him or her is in a talk that "just happens," to avoid the worker's anticipation of a planned "going over." For example, suppose a worker completes a task one day in a special, efficient way; why not say, "That was a nice job you did there; incidentally, I'd like to discuss a few other aspects of your work with you. How about dropping over to my office?"

Later, in privacy, this beginning may be expanded somewhat, and other, perhaps negative aspects may be mentioned in a tactful manner. In any case, impromptu and informal sessions are far more effective in handling subordinates than the formal, planned type, which normally cause wincing on the part of all participants. The same type of informal session can be used when an employee makes an error of some sort, providing that there is privacy and that the discussion is diplomatic and kept within the area of consideration.

Use constructive criticism

A part of talks of this kind must definitely be constructive criticism, i.e., the matter of explaining the manner in which the employee is to improve. Merely to criticize someone without pointing out how to improve work methods, avoid errors, and so on is worse than useless, since this will only aggravate substandard performance.

A good beginning might be "I'm disturbed about the quality of your work, but it's possible I haven't given you enough time and attention, so suppose we talk it over and see if we can work it out." Another type of approach might be "I know that there have been some personality clashes in our department. What's happening?"

The latter approach states the problem but refrains from assessing blame. It makes the employee feel that the rater is interested in trying to help solve some problems without nastiness or finger pointing. However, care must be exercised to avoid a heavy dose of sugar coating such that the employee is not made aware of unsatisfactory work performance. He or she *should* be told of any deficiencies in a tactful, face-saving manner that will create the rapport so necessary for improvement.

PROCEDURES FOR CONDUCTING FORMAL PERFORMANCE EVALUATIONS

1. Discuss and explain performance appraisal, policy, and procedure with the employee.
2. Review the employee's previous appraisals, devoting particular attention to established goals.
3. Schedule the meeting with each employee in advance.
4. Schedule private, uninterrupted time for the meeting.
5. Be sure of the facts; have pertinent data available.
6. Supervisors who have limited experience doing performance appraisals will usually find it advantageous to complete the form in advance. Those supervisors who have more experience or skill doing performance appraisals may wish to complete the form while in conference with the employee, or have the employee fill out the form and then compare it, in conference, with a similar form completed by the supervisor.
7. Discuss the evaluation with the employee in a warm, interested manner, being honest and objective. Remember, performance appraisal requires two-way communication.

8. Suggest and agree on methods of improvement and establish goals. To be of value, coaching must be constructive, job-related, and goal-oriented.
9. Establish, outline, and list in order of importance the specific performance goals.
10. Summarize the evaluation.
11. End the interview on a note of encouragement.

THE RATING PROCESS—STEPS TO FOLLOW

1. Review in your mind the employee's relevant past performance.
2. Review any recorded performance incidents in your file, favorable and unfavorable.
3. Review any existing written performance evaluations.
4. Review any existing annotated accomplishment reports.
5. Review the personnel records and preemployment references.
6. Complete the entire form before your appointment with the employee to be evaluated, or complete the form with the employee in attendance.
7. Allow at least 30 minutes for each person to be evaluated. The following is suggested as a format to follow.

15% of the time allotted (or at least 5 minutes) is for building rapport

- Explain why the employee is there.
- Explain the purpose of the program.
- Put the employee at ease.

55% (or 15 minutes) is to review the form

- Review the employee's work history and experiences.
- Get information, facts, and opinions from the employee as you review the form.
- Listen to the employee; get his reaction.
- Review briefly the employee's remarks (see Exhibit 1–1 in Chapter 1).

15% (or 5 minutes) is for giving information

- Answer questions or solicit questions.
- Discuss any goals for improvement.

15% (or 5 minutes) is to sum up the meeting

- Review the high points of the evaluation.
- Advise the employee of your timetable for evaluating him or her again or of your plans for follow-up on improvement goals.

GOAL SETTING

Goals are results that the supervisor and the employee wish to achieve to improve performance. Superior results are usually realized when the supervisor and the employee together set specific goals to be achieved, rather than merely discuss needed improvement. Frequent reviews of progress toward the established goals provide natural opportunities for discussing means of improving performance as the need occurs. These reviews are far less disturbing to the employee than formal meetings.

By using the information contained in the job description about the tasks assigned to the employee, the employee can be evaluated in terms of how well he or she performs each task. This evaluation, combined with a review of certain other characteristics, allows the supervisor to work out realistic goals for improvement.

The goals should not be set too high at the outset to ensure that the employee does not become easily discouraged. The supervisor should periodically advise the employee of his or her progress regarding the goals that have been mutually agreed on. Examples of goals are improvements in the following categories.

- Attendance or tardiness record
- Communication skills
- Job knowledge and skills
- Career mobility
- Quantity and quality of work
- Work habits
- Human-relations contacts with patients, visitors, or fellow employees
- Dress and appearance

Some things to remember in setting goals are as follows.

- Employees who usually work under high-participation conditions perform best on goals they set for themselves.
- Employees who usually work under low-participation conditions perform best on goals the supervisor sets for them.
- Define the employees the way they are; don't endow them with characteristics you wish them to have.
- Make the employees consultants to the hospital in their own areas of expertise. Give them the psychological privacy and personal identity resulting from recognition as experts.
- Ability is the first parameter in goal setting. You cannot motivate someone to do something who cannot do it. If he or she has potential, you're talking about selection and training needs, which can be mentioned as goals.

- You cannot motivate someone to do a good job unless he or she has a good job to do. Be realistic in your goal setting. It is acceptable to say, "Goal setting is inappropriate at this time for this position."

FREQUENCY

To be effective, performance evaluations must be done periodically. It is recommended that one be completed after six months of employment, after 12 months, and then yearly thereafter or on the first anniversary of a promotion.

Coaching should be a day-to-day rather than a once-a-year activity. The reasons for this are as follows.

1. Employees accept suggestions for improved performance if they are given in a less concentrated form than is the case in comprehensive annual (fixed) evaluations.
2. Supervisors should avoid the tendency to put off mentioning needed improvements in order to have enough material to conduct a "comprehensive" discussion of performance in the annual review.

Hospitals need to adopt a policy that gives all employees an opportunity at least annually to have a personal interview with their immediate supervisors regarding their performance and rate of pay.

EVALUATION ETHICS

If we acknowledge that supervisors must inevitably appraise employees and that there are sound reasons for doing so, it becomes important to define the ethics involved. This is true not because supervisors may deliberately violate ethical principles in their appraisals, but because it is easy to do so without thinking. We have found that supervisors can unwittingly be biased in the rating process. Listed are a few suggestions concerning ethics and the evaluation process.

- Know the reason(s) for the evaluation.
- Evaluate on the basis of representative, sufficient, and relevant information.
- Try to make an honest appraisal.
- Keep all appraisals consistent, whether written or oral.
- Give evaluation information only to those who need to know it.
- Don't accept another's evaluation without knowing the motivation behind it.
- Guide but don't dominate the interview.
- Discuss the evaluation candidly with the employee.
- Discuss a plan of action for improving performance.

- At the conclusion of the interview, make sure that the employee has no question concerning what is expected or how future performance will be evaluated.

ERRORS FREQUENTLY COMMITTED

You cannot fairly judge an employee's effectiveness in a job until you have carefully defined the scope of the job and know exactly what you expect that employee to do. By using the information found in the job description about the tasks assigned to the worker, the worker can be evaluated in terms of how well he or she performs each task. Rate the employee solely on actual performance to date, not what you think he or she could accomplish in the future.

An analysis of various evaluations indicates that while some supervisors are quite skillful in conducting evaluations of employees, a good many are unskilled. These poor evaluators tend to repeat the following errors.

1. They permit a single incident that took place just before the evaluation to outweigh previous good performance.
2. Personal prejudice and bias are often permitted to influence the employee's rating.
3. One outstanding trait of the employee is often permitted to affect the entire rating.
4. Some supervisors are overly severe, while others are entirely too lenient.
5. Unfortunately, lack of knowledge about an employee sometimes does not stop a supervisor from completing an evaluation. Evaluate an employee only on the basis of sufficient information and only for the time that he or she has been under your direct supervision.

PERFORMANCE STANDARDS

1. Does the individual perform tasks as given?
2. Does the individual perform tasks in the prescribed steps as outlined by you?
3. In the performance of tasks, does the individual accomplish the intended purposes?
4. Are the tasks performed with the frequency you expect?
5. Does the individual exercise only the proper delegated authority for the performance of tasks?
6. Is the quality of the performance of all tasks at a satisfactory level?
7. If appropriate, is the quantity of the work performed at a satisfactory level?

8. Does the individual follow the time schedule, performing the tasks when they should be performed?

Remember that performance standards are expectations of how well a job is to be done. These expectations describe quantitative and qualitative elements of the job. The supervisor is responsible for communicating the established standards to the employee.

QUESTIONS FREQUENTLY ASKED ABOUT EVALUATIONS

How can I objectively determine whether an employee should be rated unacceptable, below average, average, above average, or exceptional?

To evaluate anything is to set a value on it. In one sense, there is no such thing as a universally accepted value. Evaluations are subjective judgments made on the basis of information that the evaluator has recorded. An evaluation decision is no different from any other kind of decision the supervisor is required to make on the job. Following are factors that can assist you in a decision.

- Employee's performance versus performance of other employees within the same job and department
- Comparison of employee's pay with that of other employees within the same job and department
- Current guidelines regarding performance levels

Personality is often a major factor in an employee's failure to do a job. Should I talk to him or her about it?

It is true that personality affects performance both favorably and unfavorably. However, the point is that the employee is usually not able to change his or her basic personality very much, nor is a supervisor often competent to help accomplish such a change. If both of you together can pinpoint specific actions or behavior that may be creating problems on the job, you should talk about it. Don't ignore personality; instead, focus attention where it is needed.

Is it proper to discuss improvements in performance at the same time I tell the employee whether he or she earned a pay increase?

It isn't a question of right or wrong. The question is "Is this the most effective way to motivate an employee to improve performance?" The increase you grant at the time of the evaluation is for past performance. This is usually thought to be a good time to discuss future expectations regarding performance.

Sometimes I just don't feel like doing an evaluation. Should I push myself to do it?

No! If you are having a bad day, in all fairness to the employee wait until you are in a proper frame of mind. You may postpone doing the evaluation, but please don't ignore it or forget to do it.

Why is the Personnel Director so insistent on timely performance evaluations?

Timely evaluations are very important to employees. One of the most common employee complaints about their supervisors is the matter of delinquent evaluations. A simple way to answer the question is for you to ask yourself how you would feel if your evaluation was not done promptly when due. It is understandable that under some circumstances, evaluations may on occasion be late. Our recommendation for this situation is that both the Personnel Department and the employee be advised of the reason for delay and of when the evaluation will be done.

SOME COMMON FACTORS AFFECTING EMPLOYEES' RECEPTIVITY TO PERFORMANCE IMPROVEMENT SUGGESTIONS

RECEPTIVITY LIKELY

- The supervisor is competent in departmental job skills and wants to help the employee do a better job.
- The employee is younger than the supervisor and has had less directly applicable experience.
- The employee was hired or promoted to his or her present position by the supervisor.
- The employee's work is in good shape, and there are no unusual work pressures.
- The employee is new in the position or has just been given a new responsibility.
- The employee is eager for a promotion.
- The employee has just been given a pay increase.
- Past experience shows that the supervisor will recognize and reward efforts to follow suggestions.
- The employee knows that the supervisor will follow up on goals established during the evaluation.

RECEPTIVITY UNLIKELY

- Employees feel that the supervisor is incompetent in departmental job skills.
- The employee is older than the supervisor and has had more directly applicable experience.
- The employee competed for the supervisory position and lost.
- The employee is under unusual pressure, either on or off the job.
- The employee's physical or emotional health is not good.
- The supervisor displays a markedly changeable attitude.
- Past experience shows that the supervisor has little interest in the employee's positive response to suggestions.
- Past experience shows that the supervisor only gives the evaluation procedure "lip service."

SUGGESTED ACTIONS TO HELP SUPERVISORS IMPROVE EMPLOYEE PERFORMANCE

WITH THE EMPLOYEE

1. Clarify the work assignment.
2. Clarify the results you expect.
3. Clarify work standards, quantity, measurements, and so on.
4. Review likely obstacles and ways employees can get around them.
5. Clarify the employee's role in and contribution to the hospital's goals and objectives.
6. Review the employee's progress at suitable times.
7. Practice day-to-day "coaching."
8. Contribute your relevant personal knowledge and experience.
9. Encourage the employee to develop needed skills.

INDEPENDENTLY

Analyze your tasks. Do you need to make:

1. desirable organizational changes?
2. method or system changes?
3. facility or equipment modifications?

17

a
decentralized
budgetary
system

During a three-day supervisory development seminar conducted by the authors in Augusta, Maine in June 1979 for the purpose of validating some of the manuscript material for this book, it became apparent that the most unpopular portion of the program was the portion on budgets and the budget preparation process. Twenty-five percent of the practicing health care supervisors in attendance were unable to accurately outline the purpose of budgeting. One attendee described the process as "a farce" or "an exercise in frustration." Another attendee stated that a budget was "something one prepared so that controllers could have something to cut." Only two percent of the attendees were aware that in order to project a meaningful budget, it was necessary to analyze volume and other operating statistics. Less than one percent were able to identify more than two advantages of a properly prepared budget. Only one attendee from a decentralized-management institution was able to articulately discuss the entire budget process. The presentation on the merits of a periodic budget variance analysis and the managerial advantages of maintaining a flexible budget system was generally viewed with skepticism.

However dismally viewed by health care supervisors, budgets will continue to become chief ingredients of departmental financial planning.

In a decentralized-management institution the department heads plan, organize, direct, and coordinate. This span of control and responsibility involves money, materials, and employees, three of the primary components in any budget system. Each of these primary components is an integral part of the budget planning process. The health care industry today is replete with various philosophies and concepts on how to deliver the best possible medical care to everyone in the most economical manner. Budgeting in the health care industry has thus become a critical responsibility, not only for the Chief Executive Officer and the Fiscal Officer, but for every department head and supervisor within the institution. The industry also has many forms of controls, further emphasizing the importance of the budgetary process. One such form of control is the Voluntary Effort. The Voluntary Effort was drawn up by the National Steering Committee on Voluntary Cost Containment under the auspices of the American Hospital Association, the Federation of American Hospitals, and the American Medical Association. The National Steering Committee on Voluntary Cost Containment is comprised of hospital executives, some trade association presidents, third-party payers (Blue Cross/Blue Shield and commercial insurance carriers), and a representative of the U.S. Chamber of Commerce. The committee represents a coalition of hospital, medical, payer, consumer, and supplier interests, all committed to streamlining the many cost-containment approaches that have evolved over the years in response to public pressure for cost containment within the American health care system. The primary goal of the Voluntary Effort is a moderation in the increase of total health care expenditures. The goal is to reduce the rate of increase, not necessarily the expenditures themselves. For example, the goal for 1978 and 1979 was a two percent reduction for each year. Assuming a 1977 rate increase in hospital expenditures of 16.0 percent nationally, the goal for 1978 was a 14.0 percent rate of increase, and for 1979, 12.0 percent. The rate of increase in hospital expenses slowed to approximately 12.8 percent for 1978. The Voluntary Effort continues to challenge hospitals, physicians, and other sectors of the health care industry to do better. In contrast to the rigid guidelines inherent in most government programs, the Voluntary Effort goals reflect maximum flexibility based on a voluntary commitment by the health care industry. Some states and some hospitals will be expected to contribute more than a two percentage point reduction, as compensation for others who are not able to contribute as much to the effort.

The key point is that every hospital must use all reasonable means to keep operating expenditures and capital budgets at the lowest possible level. These objectives can only be accomplished by maximum department head and supervisory involvement.

Two other factors are also important to the development of a viable institutional budget. One is mandatory rate-setting processes, prevalent in some portions of the country where there is a public-utilities approach toward the establishment of health care rates. The other is the Voluntary Budget Review process.

Although not an integral part of the Voluntary Effort, Voluntary Budget Review Organizations (VBROs) have been organized in many states. The purpose of these entities that are organized like corporations is to encourage hospitals to voluntarily contain costs and charges for services while maintaining the quality of care. Fundamental to the achievement of their purpose is the collection and analysis of past, current, and projected data, the identification of cost-containment and rate-setting alternatives, and the dissemination of information through analytical reports and educational and technical assistance programs.

Some states have opted for mandatory rate setting, which is vastly different from Voluntary Budget Review. The Budget Review Panel of a VBRO usually consists of hospital representatives (either trustees or employees), representatives of major third-party payers, and consumers. The Budget Review Panel reviews and analyzes the budgets of participating hospitals to determine whether predetermined rates and charges are reasonably just, are reasonably related to financial requirements, and are allocated equitably among all purchasers of health services without undue discrimination except as required by federal and state regulations. Enrolled institutions pay a yearly fee for the review. Although participation in the VBRO is voluntary, some states have mandatory rate and budget reviews.

WHAT IS A BUDGET?

Budgeting is a critical function of the management. Success of a business seldom occurs by accident; rather, it usually results from careful attention to all phases of operation by those who are charged with the responsibility of managing the enterprise. With the increased interest in containing health care costs, the need for total involvement in the budget planning process has become more evident. Numerous definitions of a budget have been formulated, but common to most is the basic definition that a budget is a written plan covering projected expenditures and activities for a specific time period. A budget is also defined as a plan of what the management expects to take place, expressed in financial terms.

DEPARTMENTAL INVOLVEMENT

The Accounting Department routinely provides information to the management as well as to various groups external to the institution, such as the Board of Trustees, governmental agencies, creditors, and auditors. However, budgets are designed primarily for internal use and should be developed accordingly, with input from a wide diversity of sources within the institution. For budgets to be effective, department heads should be conscious of the benefits to be derived. Furthermore, department heads should participate actively in budget development for two reasons:

1. to ensure that their budgets are constructed in such a way as to be useful in carrying out the objectives of their departments, and
2. to direct capital and effort into the most effective channels.

ADVANTAGES OF DECENTRALIZED BUDGET PLANNING

Although the success of any organization's budget system is the ultimate responsibility of the Chief Executive Officer, all of the department heads in a decentralized-management institution share some of that responsibility. The department heads' effectiveness in executing their budget responsibilities will have a profound impact on the long-term financial success of the institution.

There are many other reasons for an effective decentralized budget system, some of which are the following.

- Progress or lack of progress toward departmental objectives is easily checked.
- New objectives for the institution or department become more apparent.
- Employment can be stabilized.
- More effective use is made of physical equipment and other resources.

- A more profitable course can be charted.
- Weaknesses in the organization or department are more easily recognized.
- Specific operations and expenditures are controlled.
- Waste can be prevented or minimized.
- The efficiency or lack thereof in an organization or department is clearly defined.
- Activities of the institution or department can be related to the general economic trend of the industry.
- Human effort can be more effectively coordinated.

BASIC TYPES OF BUDGETS

Budgets are called on to serve different purposes, thus different types of budgets exist. These are usually divided into three main classes.

1. *Capital budgets*—directed toward proposed expenditures for replacement of equipment and project activities requiring new equipment
2. *Operating budgets*—directed toward the expenditures for operating costs
3. *Personnel budget*—directed toward the number of employees and **work** hours needed to operate effectively

THE BUDGET COMMITTEE

For a budget to be effective, it must be properly developed and utilized. The budget program must be soundly administered. Budgeting is a management function, and its success depends in no small way on the support given this function by the Chief Executive Officer. In many hospitals a budget committee, composed of the Chief Fiscal Officer, several hospital administrative executives, and a selection of key department heads has been found to be a useful mechanism for coordinating and reviewing the budget program, as well as serving in an advisory capacity to the Chief Executive Officer. The budget committee is normally charged with the following functions.

1. Receive and review departmental budget estimates
2. Suggest revisions
3. Decide general policies affecting the institution and its budget process
4. Receive and consider budget reports that compare actual results to budgeted figures
5. Recommend changes
6. Assist department heads in the preparation of their budgets
7. Interpret the budget process for Governing Board of the institution

Primary responsibility for preparation of departmental budgets should rest with the individual department heads. Considerable frustration is generated when department heads are given certain budget objectives to be accomplished if they are not in sympathy with the program and have not had an opportunity to participate in the development of their budgets. In many institutions, budgets are often developed by one or two key individuals in the Accounting Department without the prior knowledge or approval of the department head. This is the worst type of budget procedure and quickly defeats the effectiveness of decentralized management and any goals of forward planning.

THE BUDGET MANUAL

A budget manual should be prepared that sets forth the objectives of the department or institution, the role of the budget in the accomplishment of these objectives, and specific procedures to be followed in developing a budget. Functions of the budget committee should be outlined in the budget manual, as well as any other roles and areas of responsibility that need to be clarified. The budget manual, which is for use by department heads, should include the following items.

1. The purpose and value of a budget
2. The department's functions
3. The functions of the Fiscal Officer in the budget process
4. The budget preparation process for the department
5. Capital budget data
6. Operating budget data
7. Personnel budget data
8. Sources-of-expense data
9. Aids to better budgeting

FLEXIBLE BUDGETING

Budgets should not be regarded as inflexible commandments, but rather as guides that assist managers in the functioning of the institution. It is necessary to revise budgets from time to time as conditions change. Not everyone advocates making budget revisions during the time period covered by the budget. However, there are quite a few hospitals that revise their projections almost on a monthly basis to more clearly adhere to changing conditions. Those who do not advocate revisions during the period place heavy reliance on the variances between actual and budget figures to locate the areas in which the hospital or department is veering from its original course, determined when the budget was originally prepared.

Two of the biggest human-relations problems in the health care field are the almost universal dislike for controls and the resistance to change. There is a feeling on the part of many department heads that a budget is a control system and will be used principally to put pressure on them or their functions. Therefore, it behooves the Chief Executive Officer to carefully avoid having the budget process thought of as being cast in concrete.

THE BUDGET PREPARATION SEQUENCE

Regardless of the mechanics, the adoption of a decentralized budgetary process will compensate the hospital for the effort by creating a more meaningful fiscal control system. It is not difficult for us to appreciate why the Chief Executive Officer or Chief Fiscal Officer might feel hesitant about adopting a decentralized budget preparation process. However, if one studies the decentralized budget preparation sequence, it becomes apparent that total control is not delegated or lost. As a matter of fact, the process is much more controlled as the budget is going through the preparation sequence, from the Chief Executive to the Governing Board.

Chief Executive's role

- Long-range planning
- Forecasting activity for key areas
- Defining program changes
- Defining new programs
- Determining capital fund availability

Department head's role

- Determining activity level
- Determining staffing level
- Listing essential capital items
- Listing essential capital construction items
- Determining preliminary income budget
- Determining salary budget
- Determining expense budget

Fiscal Officer's role

- Consolidating, reviewing, and balancing
- Establishing financial analysis priorities
- Determining cash requirement
- Forecasting changes

Governing Board's role

- Reviewing and auditing
- Giving approval or recommending changes
- Using control processes

STATISTICAL DATA COLLECTION

At this point, it would be fair for any Chief Executive Officer or Chief Fiscal Officer to ask questions such as:

1. "This decentralized budget system sounds good, but where are the department heads going to get the fundamental data for the activity levels and the staffing levels, which really support the whole system?"
2. "How can department heads develop accurate budgets when they do not know their costs of operation?"

These concerns are legitimate, because the entire budgetary system and its success depends on securing sound, basic information. If the information is not readily available from the Accounting Department, a systematic program of statistical data collection by the department heads is a solution to this problem. How many patients were treated? How many man-hours were involved? What type of professional was needed? What was the staffing mix? How many plates were used in diagnostic radiology per procedure? What generates expenses for the department? What generates income for the department? What are the productivity indexes for the department? Answers to these questions involve recording the details of each department's operation. Each department is assigned a number identifying it as a "cost center." Determining the degree to which money, materials, and people are used in different departments on different jobs will go a long way in helping to regulate the efficiency with which hospital resources are utilized.

BUDGET VARIANCE ANALYSIS

Budget variance analysis is the mechanism for monitoring responsibility in a budget system. It presents to department heads the financial results of their budget preparation and management efforts. On a monthly basis, department heads are supplied with an accounting report containing the following.

- Account (cost center) number or accountability areas
- Monthly actual expenditures charged to each account area
- Monthly budgeted projection for each account area

- Monthly variance over or under budget projection for each account area
- Monthly variance expressed as percent for each account area
- Year-to-date actual expenditures for each account area
- Year-to-date variance for each account area
- Year-to-date variance expressed as percent for each account area

Department heads then prepare for their administrative executives a monthly analysis of the major variances in essay form, as in the following example.

Account 951-243: Personnel Salaries
Actual $7500 vs. Budgeted $730

This account listing, a $730 budgeted amount for April, is in error. The correct budgeted amount is $7300. The resultant correct variance is $200. This $200 unfavorable variance is attributable to overtime pay expended during the month as a result of a 20 percent increase in departmental work volume.

With budget variance analysis, budgetary planning and control has continuing value. Interpretation of the variances is left to the department head responsible for jurisdiction over the reported activities.

SUMMARY

If the decentralized budgetary system is organized carefully, if control is exercised intelligently, and if the department heads are motivated to participate constructively, the advantages inherent in the establishment of a decentralized budgetary program will automatically benefit the institution.

18

planning for
nursing and
management
staffing

In previous chapters we have depicted various management functions; this material has been prepared to sensitize health care supervisors to their growing importance as managers in the American health care delivery system. We have given information about human resource management, labor and employee relations, decision making, payroll costs, budgeting, and so on.

If readers have gained nothing else at this point, they should know that when it comes to managing a health care unit or a health care facility, "amateur hour" is over. In today's volatile health care system, the importance of successful management and planning at all levels simply cannot be overstated. The boom years for passive management and planning are gone, and the era of crisis-intervention management and planning is quickly ending. Realizing that the future usually arrives before we are ready for it, many health care facilities, in addition to decentralizing management, appear to be ready to accept the fact that they must also have a system of workforce planning. What is being recognized as needed is an ongoing system of planning for nursing and management staffing, in order to sustain the credibility, effectiveness, and viability of an industry that is under continuous scrutiny and subject to a myriad of controls. The concern is centered around nursing and management personnel primarily because of cost, volume, and availability of these two fields in the labor market.

Hospital managers must remove the cobwebs that currently exist in workforce management techniques and must also encourage the supervisors involved in the daily delivery of health care to reevaluate their workforce utilization processes.

Traditionally, hospitals solve staffing problems on a crisis-by-crisis basis, by frantically searching for nursing personnel and management replacements within a very limited time frame. When the crisis subsides, the hospitals then frequently find themselves with an overinflated and underutilized labor complement, which is economically unhealthy for the institution. The additional cost must frequently be absorbed by the paying public. The health care industry cannot continue putting its hands into the public's purse whenever it has a problem, particularly concerning staffing. As vital members of the management, supervisors have an ethical and professional obligation to resolve staffing problems by using good human-resource management techniques.

The greatest of all organization theorists, C. Northcote Parkinson, wrote many years ago that one could identify with precision the point at which an important institution began to slide downhill—when it opened its beautiful new facility on the first day. Could this be expanded by adding "once it failed to plan adequately for the future"? In keeping with this idea, one could appropriately retitle this chapter, "Getting to the Future Before It Gets to You!"

In preparing this chapter, we had the choice of presenting either a philosophical or a pragmatic approach. We opted for both, believing that it would be more advantageous to the reader. Before getting into the details of the various phases involved in planning for nursing and management staffing, let's call the process exactly what it is—workforce planning. Let's also clarify an important point, which is that there is no single approach to workforce planning, since this process must fit the particular needs and circumstances of the individual organization. The process we are about to describe does, however, offer specific guidelines that can assist a health care supervisor in administering a suitable workforce planning program for any type of institution or department. It also offers an appropriate framework for the establishment of a process that can be used for any department within an institution, in case there is no need for a total institutional program. The theory and some of the processes were originally introduced by the United Hospital Fund of New York and the Greater New York Hospital Association, and we gratefully acknowledge these institutions for pioneering the concept.

The concept basically emphasizes that any effective system of workforce planning requires a staff inventory analysis of the highest order, one that affords you the opportunity of seeing where you are! We endorse this idea because we firmly believe that supervisors need to know their staffing situation before they can plan for their institutional or departmental situations. In the private, for-profit sector, no competent plant manager would invest or be allowed to invest in a new plant or an expansion program without adequate evidence that the labor pool in the community and the special skills needed for the new venture had been properly planned for and anticipated. But those responsible for health care institutions continue to erect new buildings and develop new programs without the slightest assurance that the facility or program will be adequately staffed.

It would be impossible as a realistic endeavor to attempt to present a program that would address all of the staffing complexities within an institution. We would like to split the broad staffing topic into two major concerns, comment on each, and give the reader some material that will assist in reaching some institutional objectives related to workforce planning.

Because of cost, volume, and availability in the labor market, the two major staffing concerns are the nursing service units and the management workforce.

STAFFING THE NURSING SERVICE UNITS

Perhaps as noticeable as any other workforce problem recognized in the health care field is the problem of "shortage of nursing labor," which has become almost a modern tradition when one mentions hospitals. The shortage has been very frequently and freely discussed and there is a high degree of acceptance by patients and the general public that nurses are relatively rare in the American labor market. Thus there is a moderate degree of belief by doctors and the nurses themselves that if the floors are in a state of confusion, it's because you don't have enough R.N.'s around! "How high is high?" seems to fit into the question "What is adequate registered nurse staffing?" The answers will reflect the bias of the respondent more often than not, and so the struggle goes on to retain what is available and to recruit what is needed on a crisis-by-crisis basis.

Efforts in both retention and recruitment seem short of success; it appears that crises will continue to be a way of life for many who are involved in this staffing dilemma, unless they are prepared to devote a respectable amount of time and effort in realistically analyzing the situation. Proper levels of registered nurse staffing in a health care institution are determined by the type of patient care needed in each unit for each shift and those on the staff (other than registered nurses) who are or should be capable of delivering this care.

The problem of determining the number of registered nurses required to give quality patient care is a real one, and we don't wish to convey the impression that we are attempting to minimize it. If one accepts it as a real problem, one must also accept the idea that it is not an unresolvable one. We believe this problem is based on the fact that very few institutions have either defined what quality care really is or decided what level of employee in the institution should be capable of delivering it! Until that definition is worked out, planning for this type of staffing will continue to be at best a frustrating effort. The whole topic is intriguing and is certainly a challenging one. Let's try to dispel the notion that it is economically sound and better for the manager to react to a situation as it occurs rather than maintain an ongoing, flexible planning process for staffing. It is wrong to accept as workable a non-system of staffing for adequate patient care because with crisis planning, no matter how you may respond, the problems become more frequent, more complex, and certainly more expensive. Health care institutions must maintain some flexibility regarding levels of staffing needed in the delivery of patient care.

Using your work force efficiently and to the complete satisfaction of all your employees (and, obviously, the patient) is exceedingly difficult to accomplish. It becomes less difficult, however, if you have a good grasp of how effectively your health delivery employees are currently being used. And we will venture an educated guess and say that from an effective health delivery point of view, most health care employees are used effectively only 60 percent of the time. Some of the remaining time is consumed by considerable overlap or duplication of work. The rest is wasted by the inactivity caused by insufficient in-service education or on-the-job training programs that restrict employees or qualify them to perform only sophisticated functions related to patient care. It is ludicrous for anyone to insist that health professionals should be expected to perform only the most sophisticated functions for which they were professionally trained. In light of rising health costs and the increasing demand for health services, it is difficult to justify that kind of inflexibility. It is also a mistake to use either artificial ratios of nursing care hours per patient day or national statistics when developing a staffing pattern. A ratio of 3.7 or 4.2 or 4.5 nursing care hours per patient day serves little purpose in establishing an effective and economical staffing pattern. Such figures do not indicate more than the count of bodies on duty and do not consider work-assignment competency levels, proper use of procedures and methods, and motivation. Neither do these figures indicate the "mix"—the distribution of professional, subprofessional, and nonprofessional levels—needed for an effective planning process used for staffing a patient care area.

National statistics concerning percentages of professional nursing staff employees needed in "acute care" hospitals (i.e., hospitals handling surgical recovery and other short-term cases) should be viewed as only a reflection of what staffing currently exists in hospitals, not what staffing should exist for appropriate patient care. The two primary factors used in making accurate staffing-pattern determinations are (1) the level of patient care required, and (2) the level of professional or nonprofessional involved in its delivery.

What nursing is today and what it will be in 1985 are questions affecting every health care institution in the United States. At the 1978 American Nurses Association (ANA) convention, the delegates decided to put a time frame on the profession's efforts to standardize nursing education. The ANA position is that, as of 1985, a B.S.N. (degree program) would be the minimal education requirement for licensure as a professional nurse. Nurses who earn an associate degree after that date will be referred to as technical nurses, as might current R.N.'s who have graduated from associate and hospital-based "diploma" programs. Diploma programs as well as licensed practical nurse programs would cease to exist. This position is being referred to as the ANA 1985 proposal. Considering the lack of sufficient clinical preparation and emphasis in many existing B.S.N. programs, the proposal may move nursing as we know it today from the medical clinical model into more of an academic model. Concern for the person, the treatment of sickness and disability, and plain old-fashioned patient care could be replaced by an overemphasis on the "stay well and you won't need to be hospitalized" mentality.

There are many critical staffing questions the ANA has left unanswered. Still, the ANA is maintaining its position that by 1985, the level of entry shall be the B.S.N. for the professional nurse and the associate degree for the technical nurse. The ANA position is basically unrealistic and contrary to not only good business management but also consumers' demands for quality health care at a reasonable cost. The nursing profession must make as its goal the delivery of health care at a reasonable cost and of a sufficient quantity and quality to respond to society's needs. Clouding the issue by misleading the profession into believing that a B.S.N. degree will enhance the prestige of nursing in the eyes of the public will, in the final analysis, serve no real purpose for effective health care workforce planning. Fortunately, nurses across the country are voicing their disenchantment with the proposal.

For years, nurses have been troubled by the many tasks they are expected to do, and rightly so. In no other field is there as great a possibility to waste the energies of professional time on nonprofessional tasks, thereby diluting the professional services to the patient. To combat the problem, team nursing is now popularly viewed as a means of solving the problem. Team nursing is a system of organizing services that are delivered to a patient. The team is directed by a registered nurse, who attends to the more professional tasks while the other team members are used to deliver services such as bedmaking, feeding, hygiene, and other nursing care tasks.

Modifications to meet both fiscal and philosophical objectives in patient care delivery have been part of a continuing process within the nursing profession for many years. Another nursing system frequently used instead of team nursing is modular nursing. In this system, patient care is carried out by one or two nurses assigned to a relatively small group of patients. All experienced R.N.'s function as module leaders, either working by themselves and giving total care to a small group of patients or working with a nurse's aide or L.P.N. when caring for a larger group. In effect, modular nursing breaks the nursing team into smaller team units. The major limitation of modular nursing is that it requires a certain number of professional nurses to implement pairing with nonprofessional personnel.

Nursing today is being viewed by many in the profession as a clinical discipline, having a role parallel to that of medicine and not subordinate to it. The belief is that the quality of care received by a patient is strengthened by a colleague relationship between the physicians and the other professionals involved in the care of that patient.

We will now consider the latest trend in patient care delivery systems—primary nursing. Primary care is to the nurse what the unit dose system is to the pharmacist. Both view their respective systems as a step toward the professional growth of their clinical practices. Primary nursing provides each patient with a primary nurse soon after admission to the hospital, usually within the first twenty-four hours. The primary nurse is accountable for a plan of care for the patient on a continuing basis, twenty-four hours a day. A primary nurse has four to six primary patients at any given time and is also an associate to other primary nurses to oversee the care of their patients when the other nurses are not on duty. Primary nurses are assisted by associate nurses, licensed practical nurses, and, to a limited degree, nurse's aides.

Regardless of the system of care, the responsibility for prudent fiscal management is still with us. It is a concern, especially to those who are accountable for nursing, which represents the largest segment of the work force in an institution. The pressure is continually on for justification of costs, meeting the multiple needs of the public, and, of course, the maintenance of a standard of care above reproach.

Primary nursing has been proven to be cost-effective by the University of Minnesota Hospitals and by other hospitals in various parts of the country. Despite the findings, primary nursing is still viewed as expensive, the assumption being that any system requiring more professional nurses has to be more expensive. Primary nursing is quite different from other systems, and the reluctance to accept it as a delivery system can probably be attributed to the limited availability of professional nurses in various geographical areas. One is reluctant to dismantle a functioning staffing system to attempt a new system, particularly when the chief ingredient for the new system is not readily available.

Professional nurses today are clamoring for a delineation of their roles. The achievement of the full realization of the professional nurse's goal, to nurse the patient, depends to a great extent on delegating non-nursing duties to other available personnel, who can and do give good bedside care. They can also order equipment, fill out requisitions for supplies, and perform some of the tasks related to the comfort and well-being of patients. A reallocation of certain tasks to a nonprofessional level will leave the professional nurse with a significant amount of time to devote to strictly professional duties. In order to implement this reallocation concept, a position analysis must be completed. Essentially, the position analysis process is a basic review of the following.

1. What tasks are being done and by whom?
2. How necessary are the tasks?
3. What is the task frequency?
4. Is the appropriate person performing each task?
   a) labor cost involved
   b) licensure or registration requirement
   c) quality
   d) quantity

The simple process of observing and recording what is being done and by whom throughout a normal work period will reveal some astounding facts. Many department heads and supervisors have been shocked to find as a result of this process that by completing a reallocation of certain tasks, more professional hours became available for direct patient care.

STAFFING THE MANAGEMENT WORK FORCE

Managerial effectiveness does not happen by chance; it needs to be planned for and developed. To develop effective managers, that is, head nurses, charge nurses, and all others classed as supervisors, it is essential that attention be given primarily to building on the strengths already in a facility. Present strengths are seen as the crucial starting point, not things that current managers cannot do. The key to the future of any organization lies with the continuing development of present supervisors and managers. Of vital concern in proper planning of management staffing for health care programs (whether existing or new) are the questions: Where are your managers or supervisors going to come from? How are tomorrow's department heads in the major functional areas going to be prepared for their future responsibilities? What strengths do you currently have within the department or institution? Here again, we advocate utilizing a staff inventory analysis that will afford the opportunity of examining the personnel levels of an institution or department before decisions are made for the future.

We have included three forms at the end of the chapter that we suggest should be used in conjunction with staff planning for the management work force.

1. Staff Inventory (Exhibit 18-1)
2. Staff Forecasting (Exhibit 18-2)
3. Individual Development Planning (Exhibit 18-3)

The forms can be modified as desired to fit the individual needs of any organization or department.

The organizational structure of today's health care institutions constantly needs to respond to both internal and external changes. Therefore, it is essential that the planning structure be analyzed periodically to determine whether it continues to meet the internal and external conditions for which it was created. As an aid to forecasting workforce needs, we suggest that the following questions be considered and worked into a planning process for staffing. Does the institution have an up-to-date organization chart? Do the management and supervisory staffs have access to it? Do they understand it? How closely has the structure been adhered to? Does the institution have short- and long-range organizational objectives? Are these objectives valid? Have priorities been clearly established in terms of patient care and service programs? Does each department have written objectives? Do the objectives call for the addition of staff at certain levels of professional expertise? How does the institution currently determine requirements for additional staff? To what extent is the staff recruited from within? What are the criteria for promotion from within and for recruitment from outside the institution?

The Staff Inventory form at the end of this chapter can be helpful in identifying the people who are potential candidates for existing and projected positions. At the same time, it will provide the user with an opportunity to review on-the-job performance, the number of years that each employee has been on his or her present job, age, the potential for growth, and other relevant data.

The Staff Forecasting form should assist the user in the difficult task of taking the long view. Developments over a twelve-month period are relatively easy to predict. However, changes and developments each year for the next three to five years are much more difficult to project. At this stage of workforce planning, one needs the answers to three questions: Will personnel requirements for the future be the same as they are now? What changes in operations or structure are anticipated? What needs of the organization or department must be estimated?

The Individual Development form should be used after the inventory and forecasting activities have been completed. It is at this point that the user should be able to plan, develop, and initiate some effective development actions. Some examples of development actions for an employee are as follows.

- Having the individual "fill in" for a supervisor during vacation periods
- Allowing him or her more authority to make decisions without having to seek approval
- Providing time for discussion about work plans and progress
- Counseling about strengths and weaknesses
- Assignment to a special project in or outside of the employee's field
- Visits to other institutions
- Attendance at advanced workshops or meetings
- Reading books, magazine articles, and papers in professional journals concerning the position

Professional competence in the health field has traditionally been identified with technical capabilities. For the future, however, greater attention will need to be given to the importance of managerial leadership and the effective use of the existing work force.

SUMMARY

In summary, let us close by stressing a short point—health workforce shortages can be real or imaginary. However viewed, the situation is correctable through the use of modern personnel practices such as workforce planning. Improved planning and managing can lead to more effective utilization of human resources and, possibly, a stabilization of the cost involved in the delivery of health care.

There are two very reliable sources for obtaining additional information related to staffing the nursing service units. These sources are (1) W. I. Christopher Associates, St. Louis, Missouri, and (2) The Center for Manpower Studies, Northeastern University, Boston, Massachusetts. Both organizations have conducted extensive studies of the various levels of staffing requirements for professional nurses. Your attention is also directed to the following bibliography concerning the American Nurses Association 1985 proposal.

BIBLIOGRAPHY—ANA 1985 PROPOSAL

Action for Quality. New York: National League for Nursing, 1968, pp. 28–43.

Altman, Stuart. *Present and Future Supply of Registered Nurses.* Washington: U.S. Department of Health, Education and Welfare, 1972, p. 75.

Befil, Catherine Waechter. The New York Regents External Degree in Nursing. *Nursing Forum* 13 (1974): 216–239.

Bridgman, Margaret. *Collegiate Education for Nursing.* New York: Russell Sage Foundation, 1953.

Brown, Lucille. *Nursing for the Future.* New York: Russell Sage Foundation, 1948.

Bullough, Bonnie, and Vern Bullough. *Issues in Nursing.* New York: Springer, 1966, pp. 1–56.

Bullough, Bonnie, and Colleen Sparks. Baccalaureate vs. Associate Degree Nurse: The Care vs. Cure Dichotomy. *Nursing Outlook* 23 (November 1975): 688–692.

Cantey, William C. Nurse, Nurse, Where Art Thou? *American Surgeon* 40 (November 1974): 615–621.

Carroll, Louis D. Utilization of the Diploma Graduate in the Nursing Process. In *Providing a Climate for the Utilization of Nursing Personnel.* New York: National League for Nursing, 1975, p. 40.

Choinski, Carol, R.N.; Carol Hamer, R.N.; Sally Hamm, R.N.; Mabel Macdonald, R.N.; and Patricia Nelson, R.N. Playing with the Entry Requirement: A Game We Can't Afford. *R.N.* (December 1978): 27.

Committee on Medical Education of the New York Academy of Medicine. Nursing Education: Status or Service Oriented? *Bulletin of the New York Academy of Medicine* 53 (June 1977): 490–509.

Committee on the Function of Nursing. *A Program for the Nursing Profession.* New York: Russell Sage Foundation, 1948.

Davis, Carolyne. Some Methodological Problems in the 10-Year Study of the Costs of Nursing Education. In *The Costs of Nursing Education: A Preliminary Report on Methodological Problems.* New York: National League for Nursing, 1975, p. 5.

Dolan, Andrew K. The New York State Nurses Association 1985 Proposal: Who Needs It? *Journal of Health Politics, Policy and Law* 2 (Winter 1978): 508–527.

Fields, Sylvia Kleiman. Nurses Earn Their B.S. Degrees — On the Job. *Nursing Outlook* 24 (March 1976): 169–173.

Highriter, Marion. Performance Evaluation: Implications for Education and Utilization of Public Health Nurses. *American Journal of Public Health* 60 (November 1970): 2079–2085.

Hover, Julie. Diploma vs. Degree Nurses: Are They Alike? *Nursing Outlook* 23 (November 1975): 687–697.

Jenkins, Glenn. 1985: Closing the Door on Nurses, New York Style. *Health/PAC Bulletin* (September–October 1977): 1–7.

Jones, Dale, *et al. Trends in R.N. Supply.* Washington: U. S. Department of Health, Education and Welfare, 1976, pp. 13, 83.

Knopf, Lucille. *R.N.'s One and Five Years after Graduation.* New York: National League for Nursing, 1975, pp. 16, 18.

Lenburg, Carrie B. The External Degree in Nursing: The Promise Fulfilled. *Nursing Outlook* 24 (July 1976): 422–429.

Lee, Anthony. Seven out of Ten Nurses Oppose the Professional/Technical Split. *R.N.* (January 1979): 83–93.

Lee, Anthony. There Has To Be a Better Way. *R.N.* (February 1979): 39–46.

McClure, Margaret. Can We Bring Order out of the Chaos of Nursing Education? *American Journal of Nursing* 76 (January 1976): 98–107.

McClure, Margaret. Entry into Professional Practice. *Journal of Nursing Administration* 76 (June 1976): 15–17.

Meleis, Afaf Ibrahim, and Kathleen Douglas Farrell. Operating Concern: A Study of Senior Nursing Students in Three Programs. *Nursing Research* 23 (November–December 1974): 461–468.

Michelmore, Ellen. Distinguishing between A.D. and B.S. Education. *Nursing Outlook* 25 (August 1977): 506–510.

National Commission for the Study of Nursing and Nursing Education. *An Abstract for Action.* New York: McGraw Hill, 1970.

Nurses, Nursing, and the ANA. *American Journal of Nursing* 70 (April 1970): 808–815.

NY 1985 Proposal Calls Again for B.S.N. and A.A. Nurse Licensure. *American Journal of Nursing* 76 (December 1976): 1893–1912.

Ozimek, Dorothy. *The Future of Nursing Education.* New York: National League for Nursing, 1975, p. 9.

Perlmutter, Beatrice. Utilization of the Associate Degree Graduate in the Nursing Process. In *Providing a Climate for the Utilization of Nursing Personnel.* New York: National League for Nursing, 1975, p. 42.

Price, Pamela. What the A.D.N. Is Not. In *Strategies in Administration and Teaching in Associate Degree Nursing Education.* New York: National League for Nursing, 1976, pp. 1, 8–9.

Proof of the Pudding. Editorial, *Nursing Outlook* 23 (November 1975): 683.

Reichow, Ronald, and Robert Scott. Study Compares Graduates of Two-, Three-, and Four-Year Programs. *Hospitals* 50 (July 16, 1976): 97–100.

Resolution on Entry into Professional Practice. New York: New York Nurses Association, 1974.

Source Book: Nursing Personnel. Washington: U. S. Department of Health, Education and Welfare, 1974, pp. 73–135.

Seven out of Ten Nurses Oppose B.S.N. as Entry Requirement for Practice. *Hospital Schools of Nursing* (American Hospital Association) 12 (January–February 1979): 1.

Simms, Laura. Two New York Nurses Debate the NYSNA 1985 Proposal. *American Journal of Nursing* 76 (June 1976): 931.

Space, M. A. Vocational Role Image, Perception of Employer's Expectations and Job Dissatisfaction in Novice Nurses. Ph.D. dissertation, Teachers College—Columbia University, 1974.

The New York Plan. Editorial, *American Journal of Nursing* 75 (December 1975): 2141.

Ura, Helen. Climate to Foster Utilization of the Nursing Process. In *Providing a Climate for the Utilization of Nursing Personnel.* New York: National League for Nursing, 1975, pp. 26–27.

Ventura, Marlene R. Related Social Behavior of Studies in Different Types of Nursing Education Programs. *International Journal of Nursing Studies* 13 (1976): 3–10.

Watson, Betty. It Could Happen Here. *Journal of Practical Nursing* (February 1977): 23–41.

We Can't Have It Both Ways. Editorial, *Nursing Outlook* 25 (March 1977): 167, and sources cited therein.

EXHIBIT 18-1

STAFF INVENTORY

Department or unit ——————— Analyst ——————— Date ———————

NAME	YEARS ON JOB	PERFORMANCE LEVEL	AGE	CURRENT POSITION	POSSIBLE MOBILITY TO	DATES AVAILABLE FOR CAREER ADVANCEMENT		
						12 MOS. OR SO	2–3 YRS.	4–5 YRS.

EXHIBIT 18-2

STAFF FORECASTING

Department or unit _____   Analyst _____   Date _____

CODE	19__	19__	19__	19__	19__
NP					
AP					
PE					

NP = NEW POSITIONS
Positions that you are projecting as likely to be added as a result of growth or expansion

AP = ATTRITION POSITIONS
Positions that will become available due to retirements, promotions, resignations, etc.

PE = POSITIONS ELIMINATED
Positions that are scheduled to be phased out due to reorganization forecast or projected economy moves

EXHIBIT 18-3

INDIVIDUAL DEVELOPMENT PLANNING

Department or unit _____   Analyst _____   Date _____

NAME	CURRENT POSITION	ANTICIPATED MOBILITY TO	DEVELOPMENT REQUIREMENTS	ACTION PLAN (SPECIFIC DATES)	PROGRESS NOTES

conclusion

Some managers always seem to have the situation well in hand. Is it because they have easier departments to manage?

How often have you heard supervisors say, "I'd love to be able to change how things are run in my department"?

Why, in the past few years, have department managers or supervisors shown such an interest in the whole management process?

Have you ever wondered why managers with a technical professional background equal to yours seem to be able to manage more smoothly and effectively than you do?

Have you ever observed how other managers seem able to sail through obscure facts and statistics and reach a decisive conclusion, while you struggle along, not able to reach a decision? Do they know more than you do to begin with, or are they just able to think more clearly than you?

The outstanding managers with whom we have been associated have some things in common, one of which is exposure to some form of management training program. The best managers, the ones with the really positive qualities, are the ones who are involved in the decision-making process within their institutions.

The characteristics of these managers can be summarized as follows.

- Strong self-image
- Success-oriented
- Assertive, particularly in matters related to their departments
- High level of initiative, particularly in proposing policy changes for their departments
- Innovative, particularly in the marketing of their professional specialties
- Consider themselves part of the management and have a positive attitude toward the management process
- Easily delegate responsibility and give authority to subordinates
- Express open concern for subordinates
- Continually encourage subordinates to accomplish personal goals in accord with departmental goals or in their own best interests
- Articulate
- Identify readily with the institution and are openly supportive of the institution

- Not coercive
- Display a genuine caring attitude for patients, families, and the public

Decisions are regarded as the bane of every manager's life. The greater the degree to which the position is structured, standardized, regimented, and fortified by rules, regulations, and precedents, the fewer and easier are the decisions the manager is called on to make. Accordingly, the Chief Executive Officer is responsible for many decisions to be made for others. This situation results in a rather strong dependence on top management for guidance.

By inspiring all members of the management staff to keep up with the state of the art of professional management, the Chief Executive Officer can help the management staff improve their effectiveness to the institution substantially.

Management effectiveness is essential at every level of the management. Each person placed into a supervisory or management position must work toward developing his or her management expertise. Chief executive officers willing to experiment with new ways of managing their institutions will find that the benefits far exceed the efforts expended.

The central principle behind decentralized management is disarmingly simple. Managers manage. When we say manage, we don't mean the offering of goodwill gestures. We mean honest-to-goodness management.

The chapters in this book are not offered as concrete principles or step-by-step procedures. Rather, they should be regarded as guides to thinking that, ideally, the reader can transform into guides for action. The usefulness to the reader will depend on the reader's ability to analyze the material and employ some of the concepts with some imagination. The reader should take the time at the end of each chapter to compare the chapter content with his or her own management situation. We encourage our readers to think about decentralized management.

The concept of decentralized management is basic and simple. A manager's job consists of planning, organizing, directing, and coordinating. Whenever supervisors or managers are not planning, organizing, directing, or coordinating, they are not really managing.

index